Young-Onset Dementias

Editor

CHIADI U. ONYIKE

PSYCHIATRIC CLINICS
OF NORTH AMERICA

www.psych.theclinics.com

June 2015 • Volume 38 • Number 2

ELSEVIER

1600 John F. Kennedy Boulevard • Suite 1800 • Philadelphia, Pennsylvania, 19103-2899

http://www.theclinics.com

PSYCHIATRIC CLINICS OF NORTH AMERICA Volume 38, Number 2
June 2015 ISSN 0193-953X, ISBN-13: 978-0-323-35664-0

Editor: Adrianne Brigido
Developmental Editor: Stephanie Wissler

Psychiatric Clinics of North America (ISSN 0193-953X) is published quarterly by Elsevier Inc., 360 Park Avenue South, New York, NY 10010-1710. Months of issue are March, June, September, and December. Business and Editorial Offices: 1600 John F. Kennedy Blvd., Suite 1800, Philadelphia, PA 19103-2899. Periodicals postage paid at New York, NY and additional mailing offices. Subscription prices are $300.00 per year (US individuals), $546.00 per year (US institutions), $150.00 per year (US students/residents), $365.00 per year (Canadian individuals), $455.00 per year (international individuals), $687.00 per year (Canadian & international institutions), and $220.00 per year (Canadian & international students/residents). Foreign air speed delivery is included in all *Clinics'* subscription prices. All prices are subject to change without notice. **POSTMASTER:** Send address changes to *Psychiatric Clinics of North America*, Elsevier Health Sciences Division, Subscription Customer Service, 3251 Riverport Lane, Maryland Heights, MO 63043. Customer Service: 1-800-654-2452 (US). From outside the United States, call 1-314-447-8871. Fax: 1-314-447-8029. E-mail: journalscustomerservice-usa@elsevier.com (for print support) and journalsonlinesupport-usa@elsevier.com (for online support).

Reprints. For copies of 100 or more, of articles in this publication, please contact the Commercial Reprints Department, Elsevier Inc., 360 Park Avenue South, New York, New York 10010-1710. Tel.: 212-633-3874, Fax: 212-633-3820, E-mail: reprints@elsevier.com.

Psychiatric Clinics of North America is covered in *MEDLINE/PubMed (Index Medicus)*, *Current Contents/Social and Behavioral Sciences, Social Science Citation Index, Embase/Excerpta Medica,* and PsycINFO.

Contributors

EDITOR

CHIADI U. ONYIKE, MD, MHS
Director, Frontotemporal Dementia and Young-Onset Dementias Program; Assistant Professor, Department of Psychiatry and Behavioral Sciences, Johns Hopkins University School of Medicine, Baltimore, Maryland

AUTHORS

BRIAN S. APPLEBY, MD
Associate Professor, Departments of Neurology, Psychiatry, and Pathology, Case Western Reserve University School of Medicine and University Hospitals, Cleveland, Ohio

ANNA BARCZAK, PhD
Neurodegenerative Department, Neurology Clinic, MSW Hospital, Warsaw, Poland

SEBASTIAN J. CRUTCH, PhD
Dementia Research Centre, Department of Neurodegenerative Disease, University College London Institute of Neurology, University College London, London, United Kingdom

BHARGAVI DEVINENI, MBBS
Staff Psychiatrist, Geriatric Psychiatry Division, Department of Psychiatry, Zucker Hillside Hospital, Glen Oaks, New York

BRADFORD C. DICKERSON, MD
Director, Frontotemporal Disorders Unit; Behavioral Neurologist, Massachusetts General Hospital, Charlestown, Massachusetts; Associate Professor, Department of Neurology, Harvard Medical School, Boston, Massachusetts

SIMON DUCHARME, MD, MSc
Neuropsychiatrist, Montreal Neurological Institute and McGill University Health Centre; Assistant Professor, Department of Psychiatry; Associate Member, Department of Neurology & Neurosurgery, McGill University; Faculty, McConnell Brain Imaging Centre, Montreal Neurological Institute, Montreal, Quebec, Canada

JILL S. GOLDMAN, MS, MPhil
Taub Institute for Research on Alzheimer's Disease and the Aging Brain, Columbia University Medical Center, New York, New York

MICHAŁ HARCIAREK, PhD
Clinical Psychology and Neuropsychology Unit, Institute of Psychology, University of Gdansk, Gdansk, Poland

SUSIE M. HENLEY, PhD
Dementia Research Centre, Department of Neurodegenerative Disease, University College London Institute of Neurology, University College London, London, United Kingdom

DAVID J. IRWIN, MD
Instructor of Clinical Neurology, Department of Neurology, Hospital of the University of Pennsylvania, University of Pennsylvania Perelman School of Medicine, Philadelphia, Pennsylvania

KALYANI KANSAL, MBBS
Post-doctoral Fellow, Department of Psychiatry and Behavioral Sciences, Johns Hopkins University School of Medicine, Baltimore, Maryland

BECKY KHAYUM, MS, CCC-SLP
MemoryCare Corporation, Aurora, Illinois

MARIA J. LY, BA
Research Assistant, Department of Psychiatry, University of Iowa Carver College of Medicine, Iowa City, Iowa

JENNIFER MEDINA, PhD
Cognitive Neurology and Alzheimer's Disease Center, Northwestern University Feinberg School of Medicine, Chicago, Illinois

MARSEL MESULAM, MD
Director, Cognitive Neurology and Alzheimer's Disease Center, Northwestern University Feinberg School of Medicine, Chicago, Illinois

DARBY MORHARDT, PhD
Cognitive Neurology and Alzheimer's Disease Center, Northwestern University Feinberg School of Medicine, Chicago, Illinois

MARY O'HARA, AM
Cognitive Neurology and Alzheimer's Disease Center, Northwestern University Feinberg School of Medicine, Chicago, Illinois

CHIADI U. ONYIKE, MD, MHS
Director, Frontotemporal Dementia and Young-Onset Dementias Program; Assistant Professor, Department of Psychiatry and Behavioral Sciences, Johns Hopkins University School of Medicine, Baltimore, Maryland

JAIMIE ROBINSON, MSW
Christ Hospital Cancer Center, Cincinnati, Ohio

EMILY J. ROGALSKI, PhD
Cognitive Neurology and Alzheimer's Disease Center, Northwestern University Feinberg School of Medicine, Chicago, Illinois

HYUNGSUB SHIM, MD
Clinical Assistant Professor, Department of Neurology, University of Iowa Hospitals and Clinics, University of Iowa Carver College of Medicine, Iowa City, Iowa

SHUNICHIRO SHINAGAWA, MD, PhD
Department of Psychiatry, The Jikei University School of Medicine, Minato-ku, Tokyo, Japan

ADRIANA SHNALL, PhD, MSW, RSW
Assistant Professor, Factor-Inwentash Faculty of Social Work, University of Toronto; Social Worker, Sam and Ida Ross Memory Clinic, Baycrest Health Sciences, Toronto, Ontario

RAJEET SHRESTHA, MD
Instructor and Neuropsychiatry Fellow, Departments of Psychiatry and Neurology, Case Western Reserve University School of Medicine and University Hospitals, Cleveland, Ohio

EMILIA J. SITEK, PhD
Neurology Department, St. Adalbert Hospital, Copernicus PL Sp. z o.o.; Neurological and Psychiatric Nursing Department, Medical University of Gdansk, Gdansk, Poland

AIDA SUÁREZ-GONZÁLEZ, PhD
Dementia Research Centre, Department of Neurodegenerative Disease, University College London Institute of Neurology, University College London, London, United Kingdom

SARAH K. TIGHE, MD
Assistant Professor, Department of Psychiatry, University of Iowa Carver College of Medicine, Iowa City, Iowa

MARIA LANDQVIST WALDÖ, MD, PhD
Section of Geriatric Psychiatry, Department of Clinical Sciences, Lund University, Lund, Sweden

JILL WALTON, MSc
Dementia Research Centre, Department of Neurodegenerative Disease, University College London Institute of Neurology, University College London, London, United Kingdom

SANDRA WEINTRAUB, PhD
Cognitive Neurology and Alzheimer's Disease Center; Department of Psychiatry and Behavioral Sciences; Department of Neurology, Northwestern University Feinberg School of Medicine, Chicago, Illinois

TIMOTHY WUERZ, DO
Neuropsychiatry Fellow, Department of Neurology, Case Western Reserve University School of Medicine and University Hospitals, Cleveland, Ohio

Contents

> Frontotemporal dementia (FTD) is a heterogeneous group of hereditary and sporadic neurodegenerative disorders affecting frontotemporal areas. A leading cause of young-onset dementia, it is often initially mistaken for primary psychiatric disorders. Based on early and predominant symptoms, different clinical syndromes can be distinguished: the behavioral variant and 2 variants of progressive aphasia; semantic dementia and progressive nonfluent aphasia. Neuropathological classification is based on protein accumulation in the brain. Pathogenic mutations in different genes have been identified. Specific pharmacological treatment is the main research goal. Meanwhile, management must focus on early correct diagnosis, symptom alleviation, caregiver support and educational interventions.

> Posterior cortical atrophy (PCA) is a neurodegenerative syndrome characterized by striking progressive visual impairment and a pattern of atrophy mainly involving posterior cortices. PCA is the most frequent atypical presentation of Alzheimer disease. The purpose of this article is to provide a summary of PCA's neuropsychiatric manifestations. Emotional and psychotic symptoms are discussed in the context of signal characteristic features of the PCA syndrome (the early onset, focal loss of visual perception, focal posterior brain atrophy) and the underlying cause of the disease. The authors' experience with psychotherapeutic intervention and PCA support groups is shared in detail.

> Rapidly progressive dementia (RPD) is roughly defined as neurocognitive decline resulting in dementia or death within 2 years. Although RPDs affect all age groups, many occur in patients with young-onset dementia. Although prion disease (eg, Creutzfeldt–Jakob disease) is often thought to be the prototypic rapidly progressive young-onset dementia, the differential diagnosis is broad and some etiologies may be treatable. Hence, an appropriate workup to determine the etiology of RPD is crucial to planning the appropriate management. This article reviews the differential diagnosis, diagnostic workup, and management considerations for this unique patient population.

Young-onset dementia is hereditary, multifactorial, or sporadic. The most
common hereditary dementias include Alzheimer disease, frontotemporal
degeneration, Huntington disease, prion diseases, and cerebral
autosomal-dominant arteriopathy with subcortical infarcts and leukoencephalopathy. Careful attainment of family history assists with diagnosis and
determining the likelihood of a genetic cause, and can direct genetic
testing. The type of genetic testing depends on confidence in the diagnosis, patient's and affected relatives' symptoms, and the number of disease genes. Single gene, disease-specific gene panels, and large
dementia panels are available. Genetic counseling should be given and
informed consent obtained. Predictive testing follows the Huntington disease protocol.

The gold standard for diagnosis of neurodegenerative diseases (ie, Alzheimer disease, frontotemporal dementia, Parkinson disease, dementia
with Lewy bodies, amyotrophic lateral sclerosis) is neuropathologic examination at autopsy. As such, laboratory studies play a central role in antemortem diagnosis of these conditions and their differentiation from the
neuroinflammatory, infectious, toxic, and other nondegenerative etiologies
(eg, rapidly progressive dementias) that are encountered in neuropsychiatric practice. This article summarizes the use of cerebrospinal fluid
(CSF) laboratory studies in the diagnostic evaluation of dementia syndromes and emerging CSF biomarkers specific for underlying neuropathology in neurodegenerative disease research.

A combination of pharmacologic and nonpharmacologic approaches is
necessary for the appropriate neuropsychiatric management of patients
with young-onset dementia. Nonpharmacologic interventions, including
psychological management, environmental strategies, and caregiver's
support, should be the first choice for neuropsychiatric management.
Pharmacologic interventions differ according to the underlying causes of
dementia; thus, differential diagnoses are very important. Antipsychotics
should be prescribed carefully; they should be used for the shortest time
possible, at the lowest possible dose

The goal of the Care Pathway Model for Dementia (CARE-D) is to improve
quality of life and daily functioning both for individuals diagnosed with

dementia and for their families or other caregivers. This is accomplished by developing individualized recommendations focused on a person's strengths and weaknesses as determined by formal neurocognitive and psychosocial evaluations. Careful attention is given to the stage of illness and an individual's stage in life, to connecting families with services that target an individual's cognitive and behavioral symptoms, and to providing education and emotional support specific to symptoms, clinical diagnosis, and prognosis.

Individuals and families affected by young-onset dementia (YOD) deal with multiple difficulties related to the altered timing of the dementias. These individuals and families are overlooked by the health care and social support systems because there are few tailored services/policies for younger people affected by dementia. This article suggests how public advocacy and interventions at the clinical and community levels can support people living with YOD, in particular the spouses, who provide most of the care.

PSYCHIATRIC CLINICS OF NORTH AMERICA

THE CLINICS ARE AVAILABLE ONLINE!
Access your subscription at:
www.theclinics.com

Preface

The Practice and Science of Young-Onset Dementias

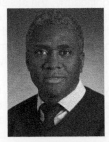

Chiadi U. Onyike, MD, MHS
Editor

*Every situation is a chance to grow
And every sunrise another chance to sow
With our hands in soil, we making furrow
Examine what you know*
—*Bambú Station; from "Chance to Grow," published in Break the Soil
(album, July 2006)*

During the last decade, recognition of young-onset dementias has become more explicit, so much so that it has become the subject of scholarly reviews, of awareness and educational activities, and of care programming to mitigate the handicap and suffering associated with the inexorable diseases.

Every situation is a chance to grow, and every dawning presents another chance to sow. And so it is that the challenge of young-onset dementia is met with a coming together of practice and science in describing clinical states and their physiologic underpinnings, defining handicaps and the needs of the sufferer and the carer, and introducing a broadening array of somatic interventions and psychosocial programs. This special issue capitalizes on these progressive developments in a series of articles that aim to reintroduce young-onset dementia to a general psychiatry audience.

Articles in this issue describe the frontotemporal dementias, posterior cortical atrophy, Creutzfeldt-Jakob disease and other rapidly progressive dementias, and other conditions besides. Epidemiology and genetics are covered. Clinical aspects are treated in articles that speak to differential diagnosis and the diagnostic process, neuropsychological assessment, CSF assays, genetic analysis, and brain imaging. Two excellent articles review the case management and rehabilitative facets. The reader will notice that throughout, the emphasis is on clinical application. We are delighted to have wide and excellent coverage of the subject, and we are very grateful

Psychiatr Clin N Am 38 (2015) xiii–xiv
http://dx.doi.org/10.1016/j.psc.2015.03.001
0193-953X/15/$ – see front matter © 2015 Published by Elsevier Inc.

to our contributors who, despite packed schedules, have contributed these fine articles.

The professionals who specialize in managing young-onset dementias have long recognized that these conditions are multifaceted—they feature intellectual decline, loss of competence, abnormalities of conduct and mental life, and psychosocial suffering. Thus, young-onset dementia is topical for psychiatry, owing to the nature of the phenotypes, the psychosocial dimensions, and, rather significantly, the skillset of the specialty. Psychiatrists, by virtue of professional orientation and their use of various heuristic perspectives in their work, have gained in their years of training the tools required to identify and treat these illnesses, manage the practical problems that arise for the sufferer and the carer, and direct individualized rehabilitative regimens.

The study of young-onset dementias offers benefits to the psychiatry profession, in the form of opportunities to investigate the physiologic substrates of derailments of temperament and other aspects of mental life.[1] In turn, psychiatric expertise has benefitted dementia phenomenology and treatment. Along these lines, it should be emphasized that since pharmacotherapy and psychosocial rehabilitation derive from the applications of psychiatric perspectives to dementia care, future refinements will require the participation of psychiatry. It is also the case that contemporary descriptions of the psychiatric presentations of hereditary frontotemporal dementia,[2,3] for example, are beginning to blur the traditional definitions of dementia, while highlighting the value of the mental state examination in the differential diagnosis. For these reasons, there is a growing recognition of the role that psychiatry has to play.

It is hoped that this issue has captured the vibrancy of young-onset dementia work. With our hands in the soil we have made furrows and, therefrom, defined a practice and science that brings together the signal perspectives of our profession—diagnosis of disease, guidance and problem-solving, amelioration of suffering, and promotion of adaptation and rehabilitation.

Chiadi U. Onyike, MD, MHS
Director, Frontotemporal Dementia and
Young-Onset Dementias Program
Department of Psychiatry
and Behavioral Sciences
Johns Hopkins University School of Medicine
600 North Wolfe Street, Meyer 279
Baltimore, MD 21287, USA

E-mail address:
conyike1@jhmi.edu

REFERENCES

1. Onyike CU, Huey ED. Frontotemporal dementia and psychiatry. Int Rev Psychiatry 2013;25:127–9.
2. Synofzik M, Biskup S, Leyhe T, et al. Suicide attempt as the presenting symptom of c9orf72 dementia. Am J Psychiatry 2012;169:1211–3.
3. Floris G, Borghero G, Cannas A, et al. Bipolar affective disorder preceding frontotemporal dementia in a patient with C9ORF72 mutation: is there a genetic link between these two disorders? J Neurol 2013;260(4):1155–7.

The Frontotemporal Dementias

Maria Landqvist Waldö, MD, PhD

KEYWORDS

- Frontotemporal dementia • FTD • Behavioral variant • Progressive aphasia
- Neuropsychiatric symptoms

KEY POINTS

- Frontotemporal dementia is a heterogeneous group of familial and sporadic neurodegenerative disorders primarily affecting the frontal and temporal lobes.
- Misdiagnoses for psychiatric disorders are common, especially in the behavioral variant, which manifests personality and behavioral changes.
- The diagnostics are based on the clinical picture, family history, brain imaging, and neuropsychological and laboratory evaluations, as well as clinical follow-up.
- Neuropathologic classification is based on the type and morphology of protein accumulation in the brain.
- The treatment should focus on managing behavioral symptoms, modifying the environment, and providing support for the families/caregivers.

INTRODUCTION

Frontotemporal dementia (FTD) is a clinical spectrum of neurodegenerative disorders affecting primarily the frontal and/or temporal lobes. Prominent symptoms include personality and behavioral changes as well as language disturbances. Frontotemporal lobar degeneration (FTLD) is the neuropathologic umbrella term for these genetically and neuropathologically heterogeneous disorders, which as a group constitute a common cause of dementia, particularly in younger individuals.

FTD was previously named Pick's disease after the neurologist Arnold Pick, who, around the turn of last century, published a series of cases in which he described the association between dementia with progressive aphasia, behavioral symptoms, and temporal/frontal atrophy.[1,2] Later, the term Pick's disease was used to define only a subset of patients with FTD with specific histopathologic features. In the 1980s, research groups in Lund, Sweden, and Manchester, United Kingdom, described patients with dementia who, on neuropathologic examination, showed frontotemporal degeneration lacking the most typical signs of Pick's disease.[3]

Disclosures: None.
Section of Geriatric Psychiatry, Department of Clinical Sciences, Lund University, Klinikgatan 22, Lund SE-221 85, Sweden
E-mail address: maria.landqvist@med.lu.se

Psychiatr Clin N Am 38 (2015) 193–209
http://dx.doi.org/10.1016/j.psc.2015.02.001
psych.theclinics.com

The clinical concept of FTD encompasses the behavioral variant FTD (bvFTD) as well as the progressive aphasias semantic dementia (SD) and progressive nonfluent aphasia (PNFA).[4] There is a strong association with amyotrophic lateral sclerosis (ALS), which is partly attributed to overlapping genetic factors.[3,5] Because cortico-basal degeneration (CBD) and progressive supranuclear palsy (PSP) also overlap with FTD, both clinically and neuropathologically, they are often considered to be part of the FTD complex.[6]

The diagnostic complexity, with regard to clinical, neuropathologic, and genetic aspects, is reflected in the attempts to develop consistent and useful criteria. The nomenclature of FTD has been subject to repeated revisions, discussions, and controversies over the years. New clinical diagnostic criteria were suggested in 2011, both for bvFTD and primary progressive aphasia (PPA) (**Table 1**).[7,8] In 2009, neuropathologic consensus criteria based on protein pathology were introduced, with 3 major subgroups: tau, transactive protein 43 (TDP-43), and fused in sarcoma (FUS).[9]

EPIDEMIOLOGY

FTD is the second most common form of non-Alzheimer dementia, and in young-onset dementia (<65 years) it is almost as common as Alzheimer's disease (AD), representing up to 20%.[10] According to neuropathologic studies, FTD accounts for 5% to 10% of all dementia cases.[10] The disorder is considered to be a mainly young-onset dementia, with mean age at onset of about 58 years.[11] Onset as early as the age of 30 to 40 years, as well as onset after 80 years old, has been described.[10] There seem to be variations in age at onset between different subgroups, with younger onset in bvFTD and SD than in PNFA, in which mean onset is at more than 60 years.[11] Some neuropathologic studies indicate that there could be differences in age at onset between pathologic subgroups, with tau-positive cases being about 5 years older at the time of diagnosis.[12] Mean duration is about 6 to 10 years,[10] and mean survival from diagnosis is about 4 years.[13] However, it is difficult to predict the course of time for an individual patient and no reliable prognostic markers are available. The prevalence of FTD is estimated to be around 15 to 22 per 100,000 in the age group 45 to 65 years[14] and the incidence is 3 to 4 cases per 100,000 person-years.[15] However, diagnostic difficulties and the concept and nomenclature of FTD/FTLD changing over time, in combination with FTD being a relatively uncommon disease, make it difficult to obtain reliable estimates of prevalence and incidence. No convincing gender differences have been found.[6,16] The strongest identified risk factors for FTD are genetic, with FTD being familial in 30% to 50% of cases.[17,18] Other risk factors have not been shown, but a higher risk for FTD after head trauma and an association with thyroid disease have been suggested.[16,19]

BEHAVIORAL VARIANT FRONTOTEMPORAL DEMENTIA

The behavioral variant is the most common clinical syndrome of FTD and accounts for nearly 60% of cases.[16] The onset is gradual and insidious, resulting in a decline from premorbid functioning. The early stage is typically characterized by changes of personality and behavior, with signs of disinhibition, loss of personal and social awareness, and a lack of insight into the present condition. Neglect of personal hygiene, restlessness, distractibility, and mental rigidity are common. Disinhibition, lack of judgment, and loss of insight may lead to socially inappropriate behavior, shoplifting, and traffic incidents. Changes in eating and oral habits, such as overeating, craving sweets, gluttony, mouthing inedible objects, excessive consumption of cigarettes and alcohol, as well as stereotyped ritualistic behaviors, are often present. Echo

Table 1
Diagnostic criteria for clinical subtypes of FTD

	1. Possible	2. Probable	3. Definite Disorder
bvFTD[a]	At least 3 of: Early behavioral disinhibition Early apathy or inertia Early loss of sympathy or empathy Early perseverative, stereotyped, or compulsive behavior Hyperorality and dietary changes Neuropsychological profile: executive deficits with relative sparing of memory and visuospatial functions	Meets diagnostic criteria for possible bvFTD and shows significant functional decline and has imaging results consistent with bvFTD	Meets criteria for possible or probable bvFTD and either histopathologic evidence of FTLD or presence of a known pathogenic mutation
PNFA[b]	Agrammatism and/or effortful, halting speech with inconsistent speech and errors and distortions (apraxia of speech) of language production	Meets criteria for possible PNFA and imaging must show predominant left posterior frontoinsular atrophy on MRI and/or predominant left posterior frontoinsular hypoperfusion or hypometabolism on SPECT or PET	Meets criteria for possible PNFA and histopathologic evidence of a specific neurodegenerative pathology (eg, FTLD-tau, FTLD-TDP, AD) or presence of a known pathogenic mutation
SD[b]	Impaired confrontation naming and impaired single-word comprehension	Meets criteria for possible SD and imaging must show predominant anterior temporal lobe atrophy and/or predominant anterior temporal hypoperfusion or hypometabolism on SPECT or PET	Meets criteria for possible SD and histopathologic evidence of a specific neurodegenerative disorder (eg FTLD-tau, FTLD-TDP, AD) or presence of a known pathogenic mutation

"Early" refers to symptom presentation within the first 3 years.
Abbreviations: AD, Alzheimer's disease; SPECT, single-photon emission computed tomography.
[a] Progressive deterioration of behavior and/or cognition must be present.
[b] Both PNFA and SD must satisfy PPA criteria by Mesulam,[80] with language impairment being the most prominent, disabling, and earliest symptom. Exclusionary criteria for all subtypes: deficits are better explained by alternative diagnosis.
Data from Rascovsky K, Hodges JR, Knopman D, et al. Sensitivity of revised diagnostic criteria for the behavioural variant of frontotemporal dementia. Brain 2011;134(Pt 9):2456–77; and *Data from* Gorno-Tempini ML, Hillis AE, Weintraub S, et al. Classification of primary progressive aphasia and its variants. Neurology 2011;76(11):1006–14.

phenomena and utilization behavior are often observed. Emotional changes such as apathy, depressed mood, and anxiety are common. The affects are often characterized as bluntness, shallowness, or indifference. Reduced speech is seen often in bvFTD, initially recognized as verbal aspontaneity with stereotyped phrases, and later as mutism.

bvFTD is the most heterogeneous subtype, with regard to symptom presentation as well as to the underlying disorder. Certain neuropsychiatric symptoms, such as changes in personality, socially inappropriate behavior, and emotional symptoms, are often mistaken for a psychiatric condition such as depression or psychosis.

Brain areas affected early in bvFTD are the anterior insula, anterior cingulate cortex (ACC), the medial/orbital prefrontal cortex, striatum, thalamus, and the amygdala (**Fig. 1**). These areas are known to be related to personality and behavior.[20–22]

The clinical criteria for bvFTD (2011) are developed in line with diagnostic criteria for other neurodegenerative disorders, with 3 levels of certainty: possible, probable, or definite bvFTD (see **Table 1**).[7] The criteria are divided into 6 behavioral and cognitive domains in which early alterations (within the first 3 years) should be noted in at least 3 domains for a possible bvFTD diagnosis. Early decline in social behavior and personal conduct, with symptoms such as disinhibition, apathy, loss of sympathy, perseverative/stereotyped behaviors, and hyperorality, are stressed. Merely fulfilling clinical criteria is not sufficient for a probable bvFTD diagnosis; pathologic imaging findings are also required. A definite diagnosis is restricted to patients with a known mutation or with a neuropathologic diagnosis.

PROGRESSIVE APHASIAS

The term PPA comprises PNFA, SD, and sometimes a third group of progressive aphasia called logopenic aphasia (LPA).[8] The neuropathology in LPA has been shown to be AD in most cases,[6] and is not discussed further in this article.

In contrast with bvFTD, in which language impairment is usually preceded by behavioral symptoms, language disruption in the progressive aphasias is isolated, or is the most prominent symptom at presentation.

Semantic Dementia

The typical symptoms in SD are an empty language, although speech is fluent with preserved syntax, prosody, and motor speech. The knowledge of words, objects, and concepts gradually decreases. Semantic paraphasias, surface dyslexia, and dysgraphia occur. In a typical case the involvement of the anterior and inferior temporal lobes is asymmetrical with more left-sided than right-sided atrophy.[23] As the disease progresses, the posterior temporal regions, as well as the orbitofrontal lobe, insula, and anterior cingulate, also become involved. Right predominant atrophy of the same brain areas is associated with a different symptom profile that resembles bvFTD. Recently, the terms left semantic variant (l-svFTD) or right semantic variant of FTD (r-svFTD) have been suggested.[24] Semantic knowledge deficits, present in both groups, contain a loss of lexical meaning in l-svFTD, and prosopagnosia and a loss of emotional meaning in r-svFTD. Some specific symptom constellations, such as hyper-religiosity, pronounced behavioral changes, and psychotic symptoms have been described in r-svFTD.[25] SD is usually a sporadic disease with few reports of heredity.[18]

Progressive Nonfluent Aphasia

The patients display a nonfluent, effortful speech with word-finding difficulties and agrammatism. Apraxia of speech is often present and this articulation planning deficit can be the initial sign of the disease.[8] Phonemic paraphasias are frequent and single-word comprehension is preserved. Early in the disease the social skills and insight are often preserved, but as the disease progresses behavioral disturbances become more evident. The typical brain involvement in PNFA is predominantly left posterior frontoinsular atrophy.[8]

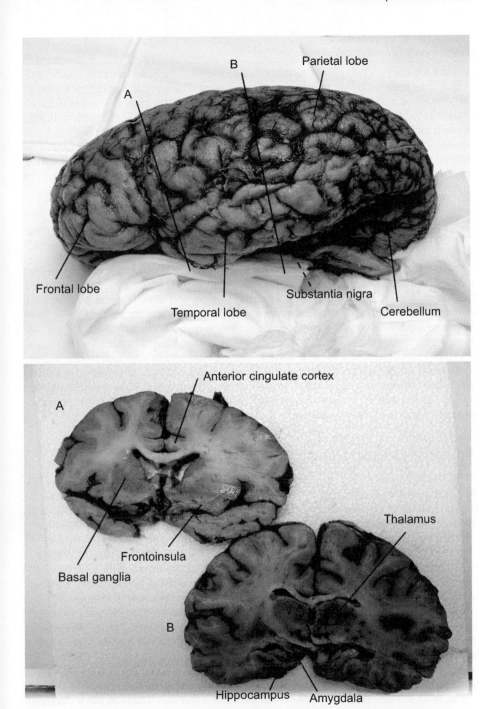

Fig. 1. Sagittal view of the brain (*top*) and 2 coronal whole-brain slices (A and B) (*bottom*). Lines A and B indicate where the slices were derived from. The major brain structures indicated in the picture are areas of particular importance in relation to FTLD.

OVERLAPPING SYNDROMES
Amyotrophic Lateral Sclerosis

ALS is a rapidly progressive neurodegenerative disease involving primarily motor neurons in the cerebral cortex, brainstem, and spinal cord. Mean survival is 1 to 5 years.[5] Some features of FTD can be recognized in up to 50% of ALS cases, whereas approximately 15% of patients with ALS fulfill the FTD criteria.[5] About 15% of patients with FTD develop motor neuron disease (MND) and, although it is most common in bvFTD, it can be seen in patients with PPA.[26] With the identification of C9ORF72 (chromosome 9 open reading frame 72) expansion as the most common genetic cause of both FTD and ALS, accounting for approximately 40% of familial ALS and 25% of familial FTD, a partial explanation for the bond between the two disorders has been found.[27–29]

Parkinsonian Syndromes

Parkinsonism, most often of the akinetic-rigid type, is a clinical feature that is relatively common in bvFTD and PNFA but seldom seen in SD.[24]

The overlapping syndromes CBD and PSP are atypical parkinsonian disorders that in many, but not all, cases can be distinguished from FTD and diagnosed during life. CBD is characterized clinically by an insidious onset and slow disease progression, akinetic rigidity, limb apraxia, as well as speech and language impairment. Levodopa response is poor. Other possible symptoms include myoclonus, asymmetric dystonia, alien limb phenomena, executive dysfunction, and visuospatial deficits.[10]

Typical symptoms of PSP are vertical gaze palsy and bradykinetic-rigid parkinsonism with axial rigidity, postural instability with frequent falls, and a poor levodopa response.[30] However, the typical histopathologic changes of CBD and PSP may also be associated with clinical phenotypes of PNFA or bvFTD. About 20% of neuropathologically diagnosed PSP cases present clinically with executive deficits.[31]

FRONTOTEMPORAL LOBAR DEGENERATION NEUROPATHOLOGY

FTLD is an umbrella term used to describe the underlying brain pathologies of FTD, which is a selective affliction of the frontal and/or temporal lobes. In addition to the presence of typical morphologic changes, current neuropathologic subclassification relies on the identification of different pathologic proteins through immunohistochemistry, in conjunction with the mapping of the regional topography of degeneration.[9,32]

In FTLD there is a wide range of severity of brain involvement; macroscopically the brain can either appear normal sized or show severe lobar atrophy (**Fig. 2**). The microscopic neurodegenerative features include neuronal shrinkage and loss, microvacuolization, gliosis, and disturbed cytoarchitecture in mainly the superficial layers (lamina I–III) of the frontal and/or temporal cortices but also the subcortical gray matter.[33] Brain areas affected early are the ACC, the orbitofrontal cortex, and the frontoinsula. White matter involvement, greatly varying between individuals, is mostly seen in areas underlying severe cortical atrophy. A specific group of neurons, the von Economo neurons, which are large bipolar neurons selectively expressed in layer V of the ACC and frontoinsula cortex, have recently been found to be selectively targeted in FTD.[34]

The term proteinopathies refers to the fact that most neurodegenerative diseases show intracellular accumulation of abnormally configured proteins that can be visualized by immunohistochemical staining. Although AD is a tauopathy and Lewy body dementia and Parkinson disease are synucleinopathies, FTLD is far more heterogeneous. Advances in understanding the genetic and molecular background of the FTLD syndromes during the last decade have made more detailed subtyping possible.

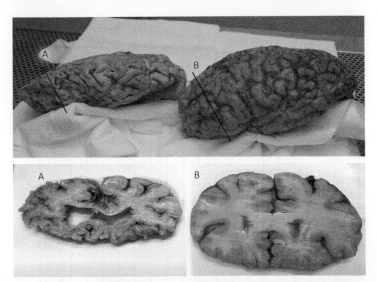

Fig. 2. Severity of atrophy and brain degeneration in 2 patients who both had clinically severe bvFTD. Comparison of coronal sections through the anterior-midfrontal lobes. Black lines (A and B) in the top image indicate the sections that can be seen in detail below. Pick's disease (A) and TDP-43 type B are present (B).

Accumulation of hyperphosphorylated tau in neurons and glia accounts for about 40% of FTLD and this was the first FTLD-related protein to be described. The tau-positive cases include the classic Pick's disease, PSP, CBD, and familial FTLD with mutations in the tau gene (*MAPT* [microtubule-associated protein tau]).

Among the FTLD cases without tau disorder, so-called tau negative, most show ubiquitin-positive inclusions and dystrophic neurites. With the identification of a protein called TDP-43 in 2006, most of these cases, as well as most ALS cases, could be explained.[35,36] According to the prevailing classification system, FTLD-TDP is subdivided into type A, B, C, or D based on the morphology and distribution of the abnormal TDP-43.[37]

A small remaining group of the tau-negative cases are also TDP-43 negative, and most of these cases are FUS positive.[38] However, despite typical FTLD morphology, not all cases can be classified as tau, TDP-43, or FUS positive. These remaining cases either show inclusions positive for ubiquitin/p62 protein staining (FTLD-UPS) or have no specific inclusions (FTLD-ni).[32]

SD and FTD-MND are almost exclusively TDP-43 positive on pathology, whereas the prediction of the underlying pathology in bvFTD is generally not possible because it can belong to any of the different types.[39] Patients with bvFTD and the combination of no family history, early age at onset (30–40 years), and prominent psychiatric symptoms often have FUS disorders.[38] Furthermore, a number of patients who fulfill the clinical criteria of FTD turn out to have underlying AD pathology.[40,41] Clinicopathologic and genetic correlations are shown in **Table 2**.

FRONTOTEMPORAL DEMENTIA GENETICS

The different mutations and clinicopathologic associations are summarized in **Table 3**. Family history of dementia has been found in 30% to 50% of FTD cases,[17,18] with a higher percentage in bvFTD than in other clinical subtypes. A clear autosomal

Table 2
Clinical, genetic and neuropathologic correlations in FTLD based on simplification of the literature and our own clinicopathologic data

	Clinical Phenotype					Protein Disorder	Pathologic Subtype	Associated Genes
	bvFTD	PNFA	SD	Parkinsonism	MND			
	+	+		+		FTLD-tau	Pick	
	+	+		+	(+)		FTLD-tau	MAPT
	+	+		+			CBD	
	+	+		+			PSP	
	+	+		+		FTLD-TDP	TDP-43 A	GRN
	+	(+)		+	+		TDP-43 B	C9ORF72
	+		+				TDP-43 C	
	+						TDP-43 D	VCP
	+			+	+	FTLD-FUS		
	+			(+)	(+)	FTLD-UPS	FTLD-3	CHMP2B
	+			?	?		FTLD-ni	?
Brain Topography								
	Prefrontal, anterior temporal	Frontotemporal (left)	Anterior temporal (left or right predominant)	Basal ganglia, brain stem	Precentral gyrus and motor neurons			

+, yes; (+), possible; ?, not known.

Table 3
Genes and associated clinicopathologic features in FTD

Gene	Chromosomal Location	Mean Age at Onset (y)	Disorder	Clinical Characteristics
C9ORF72	9p21.2	58 Almost 100% penetrance at age 80	TDP-43 type B	bvFTD, FTD-MND, ALS, parkinsonism, psychiatric presentation
MAPT	17q21.2	55 (45–70)	FTLD-tau	bvFTD plus parkinsonism
GRN	17q21.32	60 (35–89) 90% at age 70	TDP-43 type A	PPA, bvFTD, 25% psychotic symptoms
CHMP2b	3p11.2	58	FTLD-UPS	—
VCP	9p13.3	Mid-50s	TDP-43 type D	bvFTD, inclusion body myopathy, Paget disease of the bone

dominant inheritance pattern has been found in about 10% to 30% and mutations in different genes have been identified.[42]

The most common mutation is the hexanucleotide expansion of C9ORF72.[43] Other mutations are in the genes MAPT and GRN (progranulin), as well as the less common mutations of VCP (valosin-containing protein) and CHMP2B (charged multivesicular body containing protein 2B).[44] However, there are still cases with a positive family history that remain unexplained.[45]

With the discovery of C9ORF72, a genetic explanation for a large number of familial and also sporadic FTD and/or ALS cases was revealed.[27,28] The most common clinical phenotype is bvFTD with or without MND, but corticobasal syndrome (CBS), ataxia, and chorea (Huntington disease phenocopies) have also been described.[43] Psychiatric presentations, including suicidal behavior, affective symptoms, psychotic symptoms, and excessive somatic complaints, seem to be particularly common in C9ORF72 carriers. Psychotic symptoms are noted in up to 50%, sometimes preceding dementia by several years.[46,47] The associated brain protein pathology is TDP-43 type B.

The clinical characteristics associated with mutations in MAPT often include bvFTD with parkinsonistic features.[42] The associated brain protein pathology is tau positive (FTLD-tau).

The clinical phenotype in GRN carriers is often PPA or CBS, with 25% showing psychotic symptoms.[48] The neuropathology is most often asymmetric and characterized by TDP-43 type A inclusions. Mutations in CHMP2B have almost exclusively been found in a large Danish family, whereas VCP mutations are associated with the rare disorder inclusion body myopathy and Paget disease of the bone.[44]

Family history of psychiatric disorders has been recognized in patients with FTD, with an increased incidence of schizophrenia in first-degree relatives of patients with FTD.[49] Whether this is caused by clinical misdiagnoses of FTD, prodromal phases in gene carriers (in particular C9ORF72), or other shared vulnerability factors needs to be established.

CLINICAL DIAGNOSTICS

Many FTD cases are difficult to diagnose because of the wide range of symptoms.[40,41,50] Changes in personality, behavior, and speech, as well as movement disturbances, may be similar to those of other psychiatric or neurologic disorders. Mood disturbances, including apathy, euphoria, and irritability, are symptoms that often appear in the early stages of the disease and also precede cognitive changes. These symptoms are usually best recognized by close relatives, colleagues, and friends but are initially often ignored or thought to be caused by stress, substance abuse, or by a primary psychiatric condition rather than a neurodegenerative disorder. Because of an early loss of insight, other people, rather than the patient, often initiate a visit to a doctor, most often a general practitioner, company doctor, or psychiatrist. The patient's own initial complaints, if any, may also be misleading in the diagnostic procedure.[50] The time between initial symptoms and diagnosis is in general 4 years.[51]

Clinical Evaluation

Diagnosis should be preceded by a medical evaluation, preferably by a specialist with experience of dementia disorders. Apart from a careful patient and caregiver history, standardized caregiver questionnaires, such as the Neuropsychiatric Inventory or the Frontal Behavioral Inventory,[52] are highly beneficial. These rating scales systematically collect information on symptoms that may otherwise be missed (eg, delusions, hallucinations, dysphoria, anxiety, aggression, and emotional lability). Information on family history regarding both dementia and other neurologic and psychiatric disorders should be collected. A physical (including somatic and neurologic status) and psychiatric examination, including the use of cognitive screening tests, such as the Mini-Mental Status Examination (MMSE) and the Addenbrook Cognitive Examination, should be performed. However, a high score on the MMSE does not exclude FTD because this scale mostly focuses on memory and orientation. Neurologic examination should be comprehensive in order to rule out differential diagnoses such as vascular lesions, as well as to identify possible diagnostic clues indicating overlapping syndromes such as parkinsonism or MND. Axial-predominant parkinsonism and vertical gaze palsy may indicate PSP, whereas parkinsonism with apraxia and alien limb proposes CBS. Upper and lower motor neuron symptoms including muscle wasting and fasciculations suggest MND. Qualitative observations during psychic examination may strengthen a clinical suspicion for FTD. Even though most patients can be categorized into one of the defined clinical syndromes, bvFTD, SD, or PNFA, there is often a merging of the different syndromes over time.[53]

Neuropsychology

A detailed neuropsychological examination is often necessary for diagnosis in the early stages. Early changes in bvFTD may include executive dysfunction, including planning and attention deficits, poor judgment, and inflexibility, as well as loss of impulse control, whereas visuospatial skills are relatively spared. Episodic memory may be impaired, or results might vary depending on concentration and motivation, and this may contribute to a misdiagnosis of AD. Shallow contact and decreased or lost insight may be noticeable during the test procedure. Language disturbances, including an empty language, stereotypy, and echolalia, are also common in bvFTD.[4]

Imaging

Neuroimaging plays a critical role in the diagnostics of FTD, not only to rule out differential diagnoses such as tumor and normal pressure hydrocephalus but also to differentiate between different FTD syndromes (**Fig. 3**). If changes are detectable these may include gray matter atrophy in the frontal and temporal lobes, the ACC, the insula, and in subcortical structures, with variation in distribution between different syndromes.[6,54] Patients with bvFTD typically show atrophy in the frontoinsular structures, the ACC, and other structures of what is termed the salience network; interconnected

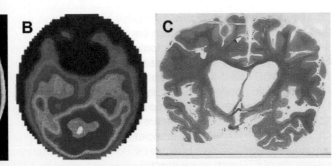

d patient was referred to the psychiatric clinic with the diagnosis of
a 4-year history of personality changes, mood lability, restlessness,
insight. MRI (A) showed severe frontal atrophy with enlarged ventri-
emission computed tomography (B) showed severe hypoperfusion in
mporal lobes. The neuropsychological investigation showed expres-
ances and difficulties in attention but preserved visuospatial skills
as well preserved. The patient died at the age of 51 years and neuro-
FTLD with TDP-43 type B.

d in the ability to respond to diverse emotionally significant stim-
ic variant primary progressive aphasia) shows atrophy of the tem-
PA (non-fluent variant primary progressive aphasia) volume loss in
gion.[55] However, in the early stages of the disease, structural im-
nography [CT], MRI) is often inconclusive or even normal. In pa-
d FTD but normal CT and MRI, functional neuroimaging such as
sion CT (SPECT) or fluorodeoxyglucose-PET may support the
gh compound B (PiB)–PET may be beneficial to rule out AD.[57]
PET tracers that specifically detect tau pathology as well as diffu-
to detect white matter integrity are under evaluation, and are not
al practice.[57]

mistry

ks of laboratory tests and cerebrospinal fluid (CSF) analysis is to
iagnoses such as infectious (eg, human immunodeficiency virus,
se), inflammatory (eg, multiple sclerosis), or metabolic (eg, hypo-
AD. Although analysis of CSF biomarkers is an acknowledged
, it has limited ability to reliably identify FTD in general or different
ncreased CSF tau/β-amyloid 42 ratio can distinguish AD from
s have shown that CSF neurofilament light protein (NFL) levels
mpared with both early-onset AD and controls.[59,60] It has recently
t NFL might be useful as a marker of disease severity in FTD.[61]

ns and Differential Diagnoses

tric syndromes rather than the whole.[65] The prevalence of apathy in FTD
n 62% to 89%,[66] and depression is seen in about 40%.[67] Apathy may be
rpreted as depression, even though the patient lacks other core symptoms
epression such as sadness, worthlessness, and hopelessness. The apathy
nought to be related to changes in the posterior ACC and the right dorsolat-
cortex.[68] However, the breakdown of specific brain networks, particularly
e network, may play a more important role in the emergence of psychiatric
in FTD than the degeneration of specific cortical areas.[22] Schizophrenia is a
nitial diagnosis in patients later recognized as having FTD, and this may not
used by a lack of knowledge about neurodegenerative diseases but also by
hared clinical features. There are several reports of FTD with an initial schiz-
e phenotype.[69–71] Several studies have addressed the similarities between
ne negative symptoms such as lack of volition, personal neglect, and social
, and the cognitive symptoms such as executive dysfunction and language
t, that are present in schizophrenia.[71]

oretation of psychiatric symptoms may lead to an incorrect FTD diagnosis.
atric conditions that may mimic FTD include bipolar disorder, depression,
nialike psychosis, chronic attention-deficit/hyperactivity disorder,
compulsive disorder, alcohol abuse, and personality disorder.[72,73] In these
brain imaging does not usually show frontotemporal pathology consistent
and the patients do not show progression over time. However, late-life psy-
sorders and bvFTD can share several psychiatric dimensions, such as
sinhibition, depression, anhedonia, stereotyped behavior, or psychosis.
ve psychiatric evaluation is called for, especially in patients who meet
possible bvFTD but with normal imaging.[72]

ept of phenocopies refers to a subgroup of individuals who, at initial eval-
ll all clinical criteria for bvFTD but do not progress during the follow-up.[74,75]
ese cases are C9ORF72 carriers, because this mutation in some cases is
with a particularly slow progression rate.[76] Such slow progressive cases
gnosed psychiatric disorders probably explain most phenocopy cases.

T AND MANAGEMENT

e are no specific treatments for FTD. Although there is still no way to slow
rogression of FTD, there are ways to manage many symptoms. A team of
with experience of dementia disorders and FTD (physicians, nurses,
ysical/occupational therapists) can provide helpful interventions and
he treatment should focus on managing behavioral symptoms, modifying
ment, and providing support for the families/caregivers. Medical, psycho-
genetic counseling play an important role when dealing with the immediate
se types of interventions are discussed in more detail elsewhere in this issue.
symptomatic treatments, the only pharmacologic alternatives that have
n to have any beneficial effect in randomized trials are selective serotonin
hibitors and serotonin norepinephrine reuptake inhibitors. They may have

and depression), treatment attempts with atypical antipsychotics should be performed with great caution. Furthermore, the risk of extrapyramidal side effects or orthostatic hypotension should be taken into consideration.

With the growing body of knowledge and understanding of the clinical symptoms, neuropathologic features, and genetic contributions to FTD, it may be possible to speculate on the development of effective therapeutics in the near future. Possible future treatment options include increasing progranulin levels in *GRN* carriers, inhibition of tau aggregation, and oligonucleotide antisense treatments in *C9ORF72* carriers. As well as efforts to develop bioactive compounds, the diagnostic methods must be further improved. A sufficiently accurate diagnosis in the early phases or even the presymptomatic phases of the disease, as well as reliable markers of progression, is a prerequisite for clinical trials.

ACKNOWLEDGMENTS

The author would like to thank Stiftelsen Konsul Thure Carlssons Minne. Elisabet Englund, Ulla Passant and Lars Gustafson are acknowledged for valuable support.

REFERENCES

1. Pick A. Über die Beziehungen der senilen Hirnatrophie zur Aphasie. Prag Med Wochenschr 1892;17:165–7.
2. Pick A. Zur Symptomatologie der linksseitigen Schläfenlappenatrophie Monatschr. Psychiatr Neurol 1904;16:378–88.
3. Clinical and neuropathological criteria for frontotemporal dementia. The Lund and Manchester Groups. J Neurol Neurosurg Psychiatry 1994;57(4):416–8.
4. Neary D, Snowden JS, Gustafson L, et al. Frontotemporal lobar degeneration: a consensus on clinical diagnostic criteria. Neurology 1998;51(6):1546–54.
5. Bennion Callister J, Pickering-Brown SM. Pathogenesis/genetics of frontotemporal dementia and how it relates to ALS. Exp Neurol 2014;262(Pt B):84–90.
6. Riedl L, Mackenzie IR, Forstl H, et al. Frontotemporal lobar degeneration: current perspectives. Neuropsychiatr Dis Treat 2014;10:297–310.
7. Rascovsky K, Hodges JR, Knopman D, et al. Sensitivity of revised diagnostic criteria for the behavioural variant of frontotemporal dementia. Brain 2011; 134(Pt 9):2456–77.
8. Gorno-Tempini ML, Hillis AE, Weintraub S, et al. Classification of primary progressive aphasia and its variants. Neurology 2011;76(11):1006–14.
9. Mackenzie IR, Neumann M, Bigio EH, et al. Nomenclature for neuropathologic subtypes of frontotemporal lobar degeneration: consensus recommendations. Acta Neuropathol 2009;117(1):15–8.
10. Seltman RE, Matthews BR. Frontotemporal lobar degeneration: epidemiology, pathology, diagnosis and management. CNS Drugs 2012;26(10):841–70.
11. Johnson JK, Diehl J, Mendez MF, et al. Frontotemporal lobar degeneration: demographic characteristics of 353 patients. Arch Neurol 2005;62(6):925–30.
12. Hodges JR, Davies RR, Xuereb JH, et al. Clinicopathological correlates in frontotemporal dementia. Ann Neurol 2004;56(3):399–406.
13. Hodges JR, Davies R, Xuereb J, et al. Survival in frontotemporal dementia. Neurology 2003;61(3):349–54.
14. Ratnavalli E, Brayne C, Dawson K, et al. The prevalence of frontotemporal dementia. Neurology 2002;58(11):1615–21.
15. Knopman DS, Roberts RO. Estimating the number of persons with frontotemporal lobar degeneration in the US population. J Mol Neurosci 2011;45(3):330–5.

16. Onyike CU, Diehl-Schmid J. The epidemiology of frontotemporal dementia. Int Rev Psychiatry 2013;25(2):130–7.
17. Grasbeck A, Horstmann V, Nilsson K, et al. Dementia in first-degree relatives of patients with frontotemporal dementia. A family history study. Dement Geriatr Cogn Disord 2005;19(2–3):145–53.
18. Rohrer JD, Guerreiro R, Vandrovcova J, et al. The heritability and genetics of frontotemporal lobar degeneration. Neurology 2009;73(18):1451–6.
19. Rosso SM, Landweer EJ, Houterman M, et al. Medical and environmental risk factors for sporadic frontotemporal dementia: a retrospective case-control study. J Neurol Neurosurg Psychiatry 2003;74(11):1574–6.
20. Seeley WW, Crawford R, Rascovsky K, et al. Frontal paralimbic network atrophy in very mild behavioral variant frontotemporal dementia. Arch Neurol 2008;65(2): 249–55.
21. Rosen HJ, Gorno-Tempini ML, Goldman WP, et al. Patterns of brain atrophy in frontotemporal dementia and semantic dementia. Neurology 2002;58(2):198–208.
22. Zhou J, Seeley WW. Network dysfunction in Alzheimer's disease and frontotemporal dementia: implications for psychiatry. Biol Psychiatry 2014;75(7):565–73.
23. Hodges JR, Patterson K. Semantic dementia: a unique clinicopathological syndrome. Lancet Neurol 2007;6(11):1004–14.
24. Karageorgiou E, Miller BL. Frontotemporal lobar degeneration: a clinical approach. Semin Neurol 2014;34(2):189–201.
25. Chan D, Anderson V, Pijnenburg Y, et al. The clinical profile of right temporal lobe atrophy. Brain 2009;132(Pt 5):1287–98.
26. Lomen-Hoerth C, Anderson T, Miller B. The overlap of amyotrophic lateral sclerosis and frontotemporal dementia. Neurology 2002;59(7):1077–9.
27. Renton AE, Majounie E, Waite A, et al. A hexanucleotide repeat expansion in C9ORF72 is the cause of chromosome 9p21-linked ALS-FTD. Neuron 2011; 72(2):257–68.
28. DeJesus-Hernandez M, Mackenzie IR, Boeve BF, et al. Expanded GGGGCC hexanucleotide repeat in noncoding region of C9ORF72 causes chromosome 9p-linked FTD and ALS. Neuron 2011;72(2):245–56.
29. Majounie E, Renton AE, Mok K, et al. Frequency of the C9orf72 hexanucleotide repeat expansion in patients with amyotrophic lateral sclerosis and frontotemporal dementia: a cross-sectional study. Lancet Neurol 2012;11(4):323–30.
30. Kertesz A, McMonagle P. Behavior and cognition in corticobasal degeneration and progressive supranuclear palsy. J Neurol Sci 2010;289(1–2):138–43.
31. Donker Kaat L, Boon AJ, Kamphorst W, et al. Frontal presentation in progressive supranuclear palsy. Neurology 2007;69(8):723–9.
32. Bigio EH. Making the diagnosis of frontotemporal lobar degeneration. Arch Pathol Lab Med 2013;137(3):314–25.
33. Brun A. Frontal lobe degeneration of non-Alzheimer type. I. Neuropathology. Arch Gerontol Geriatr 1987;6(3):193–208.
34. Santillo AF, Englund E. Greater loss of von Economo neurons than loss of layer II and III neurons in behavioral variant frontotemporal dementia. Am J Neurodegener Dis 2014;3(2):64–71.
35. Neumann M, Sampathu DM, Kwong LK, et al. Ubiquitinated TDP-43 in frontotemporal lobar degeneration and amyotrophic lateral sclerosis. Science 2006; 314(5796):130–3.
36. Mackenzie IR, Neumann M, Bigio EH, et al. Nomenclature and nosology for neuropathologic subtypes of frontotemporal lobar degeneration: an update. Acta Neuropathol 2010;119(1):1–4.

37. Mackenzie IR, Neumann M, Baborie A, et al. A harmonized classification system for FTLD-TDP pathology. Acta Neuropathol 2011;122(1):111–3.
38. Urwin H, Josephs KA, Rohrer JD, et al. FUS pathology defines the majority of tau- and TDP-43-negative frontotemporal lobar degeneration. Acta Neuropathol 2010; 120(1):33–41.
39. Josephs KA, Hodges JR, Snowden JS, et al. Neuropathological background of phenotypical variability in frontotemporal dementia. Acta Neuropathol 2011; 122(2):137–53.
40. Mendez MF, Joshi A, Tassniyom K, et al. Clinicopathologic differences among patients with behavioral variant frontotemporal dementia. Neurology 2013;80(6):561–8.
41. Leger GC, Banks SJ. Neuropsychiatric symptom profile differs based on pathology in patients with clinically diagnosed behavioral variant frontotemporal dementia. Dement Geriatr Cogn Disord 2014;37(1–2):104–12.
42. Seelaar H, Kamphorst W, Rosso SM, et al. Distinct genetic forms of frontotemporal dementia. Neurology 2008;71(16):1220–6.
43. Yokoyama JS, Sirkis DW, Miller BL. C9ORF72 hexanucleotide repeats in behavioral and motor neuron disease: clinical heterogeneity and pathological diversity. Am J Neurodegener Dis 2014;3(1):1–18.
44. Sieben A, Van Langenhove T, Engelborghs S, et al. The genetics and neuropathology of frontotemporal lobar degeneration. Acta Neuropathol 2012;124(3):353–72.
45. Po K, Leslie FV, Gracia N, et al. Heritability in frontotemporal dementia: more missing pieces? J Neurol 2014;261:2170–7.
46. Snowden JS, Rollinson S, Thompson JC, et al. Distinct clinical and pathological characteristics of frontotemporal dementia associated with C9ORF72 mutations. Brain 2012;135(Pt 3):693–708.
47. Shinagawa S, Nakajima S, Plitman E, et al. Psychosis in frontotemporal dementia. J Alzheimers Dis 2014;42:485–99.
48. Le Ber I, Camuzat A, Hannequin D, et al. Phenotype variability in progranulin mutation carriers: a clinical, neuropsychological, imaging and genetic study. Brain 2008;131(Pt 3):732–46.
49. Schoder D, Hannequin D, Martinaud O, et al. Morbid risk for schizophrenia in first-degree relatives of people with frontotemporal dementia. Br J Psychiatry 2010;197(1):28–35.
50. Pijnenburg YA, Gillissen F, Jonker C, et al. Initial complaints in frontotemporal lobar degeneration. Dement Geriatr Cogn Disord 2004;17(4):302–6.
51. Rosness TA, Haugen PK, Passant U, et al. Frontotemporal dementia: a clinically complex diagnosis. Int J Geriatr Psychiatry 2008;23(8):837–42.
52. Blair M, Kertesz A, Davis-Faroque N, et al. Behavioural measures in frontotemporal lobar dementia and other dementias: the utility of the frontal behavioural inventory and the neuropsychiatric inventory in a national cohort study. Dement Geriatr Cogn Disord 2007;23(6):406–15.
53. Banks SJ, Weintraub S. Generalized and symptom-specific insight in behavioral variant frontotemporal dementia and primary progressive aphasia. J Neuropsychiatry Clin Neurosci 2009;21(3):299–306.
54. Schroeter ML, Raczka K, Neumann J, et al. Neural networks in frontotemporal dementia–a meta-analysis. Neurobiol Aging 2008;29(3):418–26.
55. Pressman PS, Miller BL. Diagnosis and management of behavioral variant frontotemporal dementia. Biol Psychiatry 2014;75(7):574–81.
56. Piguet O, Hornberger M, Mioshi E, et al. Behavioural-variant frontotemporal dementia: diagnosis, clinical staging, and management. Lancet Neurol 2011; 10(2):162–72.

57. Diehl-Schmid J, Onur OA, Kuhn J, et al. Imaging frontotemporal lobar degeneration. Curr Neurol Neurosci Rep 2014;14(10):489.
58. Rohrer JD, Zetterberg H. Biomarkers in frontotemporal dementia. Biomark Med 2014;8(4):519–21.
59. Zetterberg H, Jacobsson J, Rosengren L, et al. Cerebrospinal fluid neurofilament light levels in amyotrophic lateral sclerosis: impact of SOD1 genotype. Eur J Neurol 2007;14(12):1329–33.
60. Landqvist Waldo M, Frizell Santillo A, Passant U, et al. Cerebrospinal fluid neurofilament light chain protein levels in subtypes of frontotemporal dementia. BMC Neurol 2013;13:54.
61. Scherling CS, Hall T, Berisha F, et al. Cerebrospinal fluid neurofilament concentration reflects disease severity in frontotemporal degeneration. Ann Neurol 2014; 75(1):116–26.
62. Gregory CA. Frontal variant of frontotemporal dementia: a cross-sectional and longitudinal study of neuropsychiatric features. Psychol Med 1999;29(5):1205–17.
63. Woolley JD, Khan BK, Murthy NK, et al. The diagnostic challenge of psychiatric symptoms in neurodegenerative disease: rates of and risk factors for prior psychiatric diagnosis in patients with early neurodegenerative disease. J Clin Psychiatry 2011;72(2):126–33.
64. Landqvist Waldö M, Gustafson L, Passant U, et al. Psychotic symptoms in frontotemporal dementia: a diagnostic dilemma? Int Psychogeriatr 2015;27(4):531–9.
65. Onyike CU, Huey ED. Frontotemporal dementia and psychiatry. Int Rev Psychiatry 2013;25(2):127–9.
66. Mendez MF, Lauterbach EC, Sampson SM, ANPA Committee on Research. An evidence-based review of the psychopathology of frontotemporal dementia: a report of the ANPA Committee on Research. J Neuropsychiatry Clin Neurosci 2008;20(2):130–49.
67. Levy ML, Miller BL, Cummings JL, et al. Alzheimer disease and frontotemporal dementias. Behavioral distinctions. Arch Neurol 1996;53(7):687–90.
68. Massimo L, Powers C, Moore P, et al. Neuroanatomy of apathy and disinhibition in frontotemporal lobar degeneration. Dement Geriatr Cogn Disord 2009;27(1): 96–104.
69. Momeni P, DeTucci K, Straub RE, et al. Progranulin (GRN) in two siblings of a Latino family and in other patients with schizophrenia. Neurocase 2010;16(3):273–9.
70. Velakoulis D, Walterfang M, Mocellin R, et al. Frontotemporal dementia presenting as schizophrenia-like psychosis in young people: clinicopathological series and review of cases. Br J Psychiatry 2009;194(4):298–305.
71. Harciarek M, Malaspina D, Sun T, et al. Schizophrenia and frontotemporal dementia: shared causation? Int Rev Psychiatry 2013;25(2):168–77.
72. Pose M, Cetkovich M, Gleichgerrcht E, et al. The overlap of symptomatic dimensions between frontotemporal dementia and several psychiatric disorders that appear in late adulthood. Int Rev Psychiatry 2013;25(2):159–67.
73. Manes F. Psychiatric conditions that can mimic early behavioral variant frontotemporal dementia: the importance of the new diagnostic criteria. Curr Psychiatry Rep 2012;14(5):450–2.
74. Hornberger M, Shelley BP, Kipps CM, et al. Can progressive and non-progressive behavioural variant frontotemporal dementia be distinguished at presentation? J Neurol Neurosurg Psychiatry 2009;80(6):591–3.
75. Davies RR, Kipps CM, Mitchell J, et al. Progression in frontotemporal dementia: identifying a benign behavioral variant by magnetic resonance imaging. Arch Neurol 2006;63(11):1627–31.

76. Gomez-Tortosa E, Serrano S, de Toledo M, et al. Familial benign frontotemporal deterioration with C9ORF72 hexanucleotide expansion. Alzheimers Dement 2014;10(5 Suppl):S284–9.
77. D'Alton S, Lewis J. Therapeutic and diagnostic challenges for frontotemporal dementia. Front Aging Neurosci 2014;6:204.
78. Boxer AL, Knopman DS, Kaufer DI, et al. Memantine in patients with frontotemporal lobar degeneration: a multicentre, randomised, double-blind, placebo-controlled trial. Lancet Neurol 2013;12(2):149–56.
79. Vercelletto M, Boutoleau-Bretonniere C, Volteau C, et al. Memantine in behavioral variant frontotemporal dementia: negative results. J Alzheimers Dis 2011;23(4): 749–59.
80. Mesulam MM. Primary progressive aphasia. Ann Neurol 2001;49(4):425–32.

Posterior Cortical Atrophy
An Atypical Variant of Alzheimer Disease

Aida Suárez-González, PhD*, Susie M. Henley, PhD, Jill Walton, MSc,
Sebastian J. Crutch, PhD

KEYWORDS

- Neuropsychiatry manifestations (NPM) • PCA • Young-onset dementia • Apathy
- Depression • Posterior atrophy • Visual impairment • Peer support

KEY POINTS

- Patients with posterior cortical atrophy (PCA) present an atypical phenotype different from typical (amnesic) Alzheimer disease (AD) in that it is characterized by midlife onset, progressive visual dysfunction, and focal posterior (occipital and parietal) atrophy; hence, neuropsychiatric phenomena also differ from those of typical AD.
- The neuropsychiatric profile in PCA is often overlooked and merits attention because of its impact on the patients' quality of life and prognostic implications.
- Apathy, anxiety, depression, and irritability are the most common neuropsychiatric manifestations (NPM) in PCA.
- Neuropsychiatric examination is an essential tool for discriminating PCA caused by AD and dementia with Lewy bodies.
- Focused interviewing targeting NPM must be included in the clinical interview, and validated neuropsychiatric scales should be added to neuropsychological assessments.
- Individualized therapy including cognitive-behavioral therapy is valuable in PCA.
- Support groups are powerful intervention tools for patients and families.

INTRODUCTION

Posterior cortical atrophy (PCA) is a clinical syndrome characterized by progressive loss of visual processing and other posterior brain functions (including reading,

Disclosures: This work was undertaken at UCLH/UCL, which received a proportion of funding from the Department of Health's NIHR Biomedical Research Centres funding scheme. The Dementia Research Centre is an Alzheimer's Research UK Coordinating Centre. A. Suárez-González was supported by a Dunhill Medical Trust grant (R337/0214). This work was supported by an Alzheimer's Research UK Senior Research Fellowship and ESRC/NIHR grant (ES/K006711/1) to S. Crutch. This work was supported by the NIHR Queen Square Dementia Biomedical Research Unit.
Dementia Research Centre, Department of Neurodegenerative Disease, UCL Institute of Neurology, University College London, Queen Square, London WC1N 3BG, UK
* Correspondence author. Dementia Research Centre, Box 16, National Hospital for Neurology and Neurosurgery, Queen Square, London WC1N 3BG, UK.
E-mail address: aida.gonzalez@ucl.ac.uk

Psychiatr Clin N Am 38 (2015) 211–220
http://dx.doi.org/10.1016/j.psc.2015.01.009
0193-953X/15/$ – see front matter © 2015 Elsevier Inc. All rights reserved.

Abbreviations	
AD	Alzheimer disease
CBT	Cognitive-behavioral therapy
DLB	Dementia with Lewy bodies
LOAD	Late-onset Alzheimer disease
NPM	Neuropsychiatry manifestations
PCA	Posterior cortical atrophy
PCA-AD	Posterior cortical atrophy–Alzheimer disease
PCA-DLB	Posterior cortical atrophy–dementia with Lewy bodies
VH	Visual hallucinations
YOAD	Young-onset Alzheimer disease

calculation, and navigational orientation) and atrophy of the parietal, occipital, and occipitotemporal cortices.[1] Alzheimer disease (AD) is the most common underlying pathologic state (up to 78% of patients with PCA having pathological confirmed AD[1]) with alternative causes including dementia with Lewy bodies (DLB), subcortical gliosis, corticobasal degeneration, and prion-associated disease.[1–4] There are no epidemiologic studies of PCA, but it has been estimated that PCA may account for 5% to 10% of young-onset AD (YOAD) presentations.[5] Age at onset is usually lower in PCA than in typical (amnesic) AD, with most patients with PCA experiencing their first symptoms in their 50s or early 60s.[6,7]

Patients with PCA report difficulties in reading, driving, navigating, and identifying objects.[1,6–8] In many senses these patients behave as if blind, regardless of their preserved visual acuity and absence of ophthalmologic impairment. Very often they are referred by ophthalmologists, as visual difficulties are commonly their first and main complaint. Deterioration in other cognitive domains comes over time, degrading posterior functions, such praxis, calculation, and spelling first, whereas episodic memory, insight, and anterior functions (such as attention and executive functions) are relatively preserved until later in the disease. Although research on the neurologic, cognitive, and neuroimaging characteristics of PCA have increased during the last 2 decades, the neuropsychiatric manifestations (NPM) have received little attention and are consequently poorly characterized. More than 80% of patients with typical AD have some kind of neuropsychiatric disorder over the course of the disease[9]; these rates are even higher in DLB.[10] In short, NPM have proved to be highly prevalent in patients with dementia, are a domain of great complexity, and have important implications for diagnosis, treatment, and prognosis.[10–14] Studying NPM in atypical phenotypes of AD is particularly challenging because the prevalence of these forms is low and missed diagnosis common. Furthermore, in the case of syndromes in which specific clinical features are particularly salient and striking (such as visual disturbances in PCA), other regular features (eg, depression or delusions) may be overlooked.

NEUROPSYCHIATRIC MANIFESTATIONS AND CLINICAL PICTURE

In this review, the authors examine the evidence concerning similarities and differences in the patterns of NPM expressed by individuals with PCA and typical AD. One pertinent factor is the younger age at onset of PCA compared with typical AD. The data regarding the prevalence of NPM in YOAD (cases with onset before 65 years of age) and late-onset AD (LOAD) are equivocal, as some studies report a higher prevalence of NPM in YOAD and others in LOAD.[12,15–17] The problem of interpretation is that these studies generally have small samples, and the YOAD samples are likely to include other atypical AD phenotypes (such as frontal-variant AD, which mimics frontotemporal dementia, and logopenic progressive aphasia, a form of primary progressive aphasia). Recent longitudinal studies, which have enrolled larger numbers, have described lower prevalence of depression, anxiety, apathy, and irritability in younger compared with older AD.[12,16] However, the data are ambiguous because these studies specify a diagnosis of AD but do not distinguish between typical and atypical phenotypes. In the authors' opinion, it is premature to conclude that patients with PCA have a lower frequency of NPM symptoms than patients with LOAD.

In this article, the authors divide NPM into 2 major domains[1]: emotional features, consisting of apathy, depression, anxiety, euphoria, and irritability, and[2] psychotic features, including hallucinations, delusions, and delusional misidentifications.

Emotional Features

The only study to date examining the NPM of PCA reported apathy (60%), anxiety (55%), depression (45%), and irritability (35%) as the most common NPM in PCA.[18] The study found differences in the rates of anxiety between PCA and AD (55% PCA, 15% AD, $P<.01$); there were no differences in cognition, age, education, illness duration, or severity between anxious and nonanxious patients with PCA. In a forthcoming study done by the authors' group, the neuropsychiatric profile did not differ between 28 subjects with PCA and 34 with AD (matched by age, disease severity, and illness duration) (Suarez-Gonzalez A, Crutch S, Franco E, and colleagues, unpublished data, 2015).[19] Depression, irritability, anxiety, and apathy were the most frequent symptoms in the PCA and AD groups. The authors found age-related differences in the levels of anxiety, with patients with YOAD having more than their LOAD counterparts, whereas there were no differences between young- and late-onset PCA. Taken together, the findings from these two studies are similar, the exception being that rates of anxiety in the authors' AD group (55%) are higher than rates in the other study (15%).

Apathy and depression were the only emotional features reported in the PCA literature until recently.[18] Apathy is a disorder of the initiation, intensity, and persistence of goal-directed behavior and is the most common NPM in YOAD.[12,14,16,19,20] It is the most persistent and frequent NPM in all the stages of typical AD,[14] also the most common in PCA[18] in one study, and the next more common after depression and irritability in another (Suarez-Gonzalez A, Crutch S, Franco E, and colleagues, unpublished data, 2015).[19] Shakespeare and colleagues[21] have suggested that apathy in PCA may be less severe than in amnesic AD, based on their analysis of scores derived from the Cambridge Behavioral Inventory-Revised. The authors' most recent data replicate this finding (Suarez-Gonzalez A, Crutch S, Franco E, and colleagues, unpublished data, 2015).[19] Although this observation is not yet confirmed, it is consistent with other data showing associations of apathy in AD with dysfunction in the anterior cingulate and in fronto-subcortical circulates,[22,23] all cortical regions having less degeneration in PCA than in AD.

The prevalence of depressive symptoms in AD can amount to 30% to 79%,[24–26] making it one of the most common NPM in PCA and amnesic phenotypes (Suarez-Gonzalez A, Crutch S, Franco E, and colleagues, unpublished data, 2015).[18,19] It should be noted, however, that there are very few studies of this in PCA. A case report has described PCA presenting first as treatment-resistant major depression.[27] Another study found patients with PCA to be more prone to having depression than patients with amnesic AD.[6] The conclusion was that depression in PCA reflects a reaction stemming from the patients' awareness of their handicaps, which is consistent with these patients' general preservation of insight and executive functions. This argument that greater insight in PCA regularly results in depressive reactions is not new, but the authors are not yet convinced of this explanation. First, there is a high frequency of depression in AD; that association is well established in the amnesic phenotype whereby loss of insight is common. Although the relation between depression and risk for later development of dementia is still unclear, both disorders seem to share common neuropathologic mechanisms involving modulation of neurotransmitters.[28–30] Secondly, the fact that patients with PCA seem to present with similar rates of depression as those with typical AD (in studies measuring with tools such as the Neuropsychiatric Inventory) argues against a direct (or primary) influence of insight in the development of depressive symptoms. It is, however, possible that the nature of depressive symptoms varies in individuals with PCA and other AD phenotypes, as such insight might be indirectly involved in its modulation. Thirdly, white matter lesions may deregulate mood in late life[31] and become an added variable contributing to depressive symptoms in AD syndromes. In light of these findings, it seems reasonable at least to consider that depression in PCA has a multifactorial origin.

Psychotic Features: Hallucinations and Delusional Misidentification

Visual hallucinations (VH) have been described in up to 5% to 31% of patients with PCA.[1,3,7] In a large case series, Josephs and colleagues[3] found that 13 out of 59 (22%) patients with PCA exhibited VH, and all patients met the criteria for DLB.[10] This finding is consistent with findings reported by McMonagle and colleagues[7] in whose sample 6 out of 19 patients presented VH, and 5 of the 6 patients were diagnosed with DLB. Furuya and colleagues[32] also described a patient with frequent VH in the absence of parkinsonism at the time of assessment, 3 years after disease onset; but there was no pathologic information in this case. In the authors' own sample, the 3 patients who presented with VH also met the criteria for probable DLB (3 out of 28); these individuals accounted for 10% of the total sample (Suarez-Gonzalez A, Crutch S, Franco E, and colleagues, unpublished data, 2015).[19] In light of these studies, it seems that VH in PCA usually occurs in individuals fulfilling the criteria for DLB. These estimates of the relative prevalence of PCA-DLB from clinical studies are largely consistent with rates of DLB determined in the few pathologic series of PCA (22.0% [2 out of 9 autopsies][1]; 9.5% [2 out of 21 autopsies][2]). In the study by Tang-Wai and colleagues,[1] 2 patients presenting Lewy body pathology developed illness at 65 and 58 years of age and had the disease for 10 and 14 years, respectively.

Establishing the frequency of VH in PCA is important for the differential diagnosis of PCA caused by AD or DLB, as VH are a major feature of the DLB diagnostic criteria.[10] The distinction is also important for prognosis and treatment, given that the interventions for DLB and AD differ.

The posterior nature of atrophy in PCA has been considered as a possible source of VH. However, posterior atrophy in PCA is pronounced and VH unusual, whereas in DLB there is less posterior atrophy and VH are much more frequent. Therefore, other factors besides posterior atrophy must be sought. Considering anatomic associations, a VBM study of VH in PCA[3] showed that patients with PCA with VH had more atrophy than those without VH in the primary visual cortex but also in subcortical structures (lentiform nuclei, thalamus, basal forebrain and midbrain). Also, cholinergic and monoaminergic dysfunction in AD and DLB may be contributors to the NPM in these diseases.[13,33] It remains unsettled whether the pronounced occipital atrophy observed in PCA contributes to the appearance of VH. So too remains unknown whether there are qualitative differences in the nature of hallucinations experienced by PCA-AD compared with PCA-DLB.

To the authors' knowledge, the patient reported by Yoshida and colleagues[34] and presenting with a mirror sign is the only case of a delusional misidentification in

PCA in the literature. The authors also examined delusions and delusional misidenti-fications in their study, including frequency and composition, and did not find differ-ences between PCA and amnesic AD (Suarez-Gonzalez A, Crutch S, Franco E, and colleagues, unpublished data, 2015).[19]

TREATMENT AND THERAPEUTIC APPROACH
Individualized Therapy and Support

As with NPM in PCA, there has been very little empirical work on psychotherapeutic approaches to mental health problems in PCA. There is one study evaluating the effect of a tailored psychoeducation program for patients with PCA and their caregivers, which reduced anxiety in the caregivers.[35] This dearth of research is caused in part by the rarity of the syndrome but also a tendency in the field to use *dementia* as an all-encompassing term (or even as a synonym for AD), which overlooks the different pathologic types and phenotypes and the fact that different types of dementia differ in the care needs. There is growing evidence of the effectiveness of psychotherapeutic interventions for mental health problems in dementia (such as cognitive-behavioral therapy [CBT] for anxiety and depression) and for caregivers of people with dementia (eg,[36,37]), although most studies focus on late-onset dementia and many do not specify the subtype of dementia. There is also a slowly growing body of evidence about the specific needs of people with young-onset dementia, but these tend to focus on young-onset AD (eg,[38]) and sometimes frontotemporal dementia (eg,[39]). Although it seems likely that some of the issues identified as important for young-onset dementia will apply regardless of phenotype (for example, disruption of the life cycle, having young children, feeling out of place in services designed for people older than 65 years), the nature of PCA also brings with it unique challenges that are not necessarily found in other presentations.

Experience from the psychological therapies service attached to the Specialist Cognitive Disorders clinic at the National Hospital for Neurology and Neurosurgery suggests that this is the case. There are several themes that arise repeatedly in thera-peutic sessions with patients with PCA that seem less prominent for other presenta-tions. One is the comparatively very early loss of privacy and independence in PCA: at a point at which people with amnesic AD or an aphasic condition such as nonfluent primary progressive aphasia[40] can still pass a driving test, read correspondence, and choose what to wear, for example, patients with PCA are likely to be unable to exercise these skills and opportunities while being acutely aware of their loss and dependence on those around them for these functions. Of course these skills are eventually affected in typical AD; the key difference being that they are affected disproportionately and earlier in PCA. Many patients report feeling guilty, angry, frustrated, and low at becoming so dependent on others; many patients withdraw from social activities, not because they are unable to participate but because they wish to avoid asking others for the help they need to do so. A corollary of this is the frustration often reported by families who understand dementia to be a memory disease and cannot comprehend why their loved one can no longer reach out and pick up a mug of tea (a common dif ficulty in PCA when patients lose the visuospatial skills to map where external items are in relation to themselves and to coordinate their own movements toward those items) but can still converse articulately about current affairs and remember shopping lists. Understandably these misperceptions can lead to conflict and are a source, therefore, of psychological distress in patients and their caregivers. Attendees of this service routinely complete the Depression Anxiety Stress Scales 21 mood questionnaire (http://www2.psy.unsw.edu.au/groups/dass); both patients with PCA and their caregivers frequently check items putting them in the mild to severe ranges for depression, anxiety, or stress, although the authors have insufficient data to determine what might influence individual differences in these scores for this population.

In the authors' experience, much of the work centers on psychoeducation about PCA (for both patients and carers/families); relationship to help,[41] particularly thinking about the patients' past help-giving and help-receiving in the context of their family; and taking a CBT approach in identifying unhelpful patterns of thoughts, feelings, and behavior by applying techniques, such as thought-challenging, positive data logs, and relaxation training, to develop more useful alternatives. It should be noted that, in the authors' experience, CBT techniques can be used with very little modification with patients with PCA, who are usually capable of holding, understanding, and manipulating information in the mind but may need assistance with written materials. It seems likely that other psychotherapeutic techniques would also be helpful with little modification.

Support Groups

When we consider therapeutic approaches that may be beneficial for people with PCA, we must acknowledge that people living with a diagnosis of PCA generally do so in the community, supported by informal caregivers typically made up of spouses, relatives, friends, and neighbors. The pressures of understanding and managing a relatively rare diagnosis can produce negative mental and physical consequences for both the person and his or her caregivers. Research shows that caregivers of younger people with dementia have higher levels of burden than their older counterparts, even when matched for severity of dementia and behavioral disturbance.[42]

Support groups have a constructive role to play in offering people the opportunity to acknowledge their diagnosis and its consequences alongside peers in a similar position who understand their predicament. Support groups provide a space in which to share one's story, among listeners who understand and empathize, and, therefore, provide a setting in which acceptance of a diagnosis and the requisite adaptations is facilitated.

Quite apart from the social and emotional benefits of participating, disease-specific support groups allow for the exchange of valuable professional and personal information and advice—gateways to understanding and sharing that enable people to cope better and for longer. Education and skills development, together with preparing people for the future, recognizing common struggles, and being able to have conversations about life-changing circumstances in a safe environment, can all contribute to a reduction in fear, anxiety, and isolation.

In a review and assessment of the data, Chu and colleagues[43] examined the effectiveness of support groups for caregivers of people with dementia. They examined the impact of mutual support groups, psychoeducational, and educational support groups alike. Outcome indicators measured psychological well-being, depression, burden, and social function. Attendance at support groups was positively associated with caregivers' psychological well-being and social function, although further work is required to identify how to maximize support group effectiveness.

Support groups typically take the form of a physical meeting in a prearranged venue but can also extend to supportive networks across telephone, Internet, and social media platforms, as well as provide the opportunity for people to develop one-to-one peer relationships that are continued outside of the formal meetings. Webinar and Skype (Microsoft Corporation, Redmond, WA) technology allow group members who would otherwise be unable to attend a meeting to join the event and benefit from virtual participation.

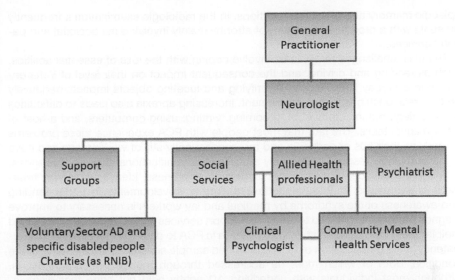

Fig. 1. Pyramid of resources available for patients with PCA. Allied Health professionals: professionals involved in clinical care distinct from the medical and nursing professions, eg. Speech therapists, physiotherapists, occupational therapists, etc...RNIB: in UK, Royal National Institute of Blind People.

The authors' experience running the Posterior Cortical Atrophy Support Group (founded in 2007) is that patients with PCA and their families and friends benefit from the support of the skilled nurse adviser and coordinator attached to the group. As well as facilitating group meetings, the nurse adviser is available to answer disease-specific queries by phone or e-mail and follow up group members on a one-to-one basis.

Distinct from the personal and individual benefit to group members, the support group also fulfills an advocacy role on behalf of its members by raising awareness and representing the needs of people within the group by contributing to debates and discussions at a more strategic level. For example, a recent support group initiative sought to raise awareness of PCA at a House of Lords parliamentary event to which key professionals and political stakeholders across a range of social and care provider networks were invited. Group members themselves can also play a complementary role in this function. People from across the United Kingdom and indeed globally are accessing the authors' support group services in the absence of local alternatives, and the authors have seen an increase in membership in the past 12 to 18 months. Web traffic is also increasing, and the increasing number of personal contacts made to the support group coordinator is a factor that further validates the role and value of support groups for people with this diagnosis. A chart illustrating services available for patients with PCA is shown in **Fig. 1,** and details about the group can be accessed at: http://www.ucl.ac.uk/drc/pcasupport.

SUMMARY

In summary, PCA is a syndrome that can be identified in the clinical setting by its most prominent features: insidious onset (often younger than 65 years) with progressive loss of visual, praxis, calculation, and navigation skills compared with relatively spared episodic memory and executive functions. In the radiologic examination it frequently presents with a pronounced pattern of atrophy mainly involving the occipital and parietal cortices.

The main challenges for patients involve coping with the loss of essential abilities, such as reading and driving, and the consequent impact on their level of independence in everyday life. Difficulty identifying and locating objects impacts negatively on their relationship with the environment. Increasing apraxia also leads to difficulties using cutlery, putting clothes on, grooming, writing, using computers, and a host of other manual tasks. The fact that most people with PCA experience these problems as early as their 50s or early 60s and are consequently still of working age and have significant family responsibilities only amplifies the ramifications of these challenges.

The last 2 decades have brought increasing awareness, identification, and treatment of symptoms in PCA. Nonetheless, further developments in understanding and awareness of the syndrome by medical and lay workers is necessary to improve diagnosis and treatment and to enhance support services for individuals with PCA and their families. The main limitations on research in PCA to date have been a lack of consistency in the classification of PCA and limited sample sizes owing to the rarity of the condition, both of which must be addressed through multicenter collaborations. Although most individuals with underlying AD rightly hold out hope that disease-modifying treatments for typical AD will be equally effective in PCA, dedicated trials will also be required to assess the usefulness of pharmacologic and nonpharmacologic interventions in PCA.

REFERENCES

1. Tang-Wai DF, Graff-Radford NR, Boeve BF, et al. Clinical, genetic, and neuropathologic characteristics of posterior cortical atrophy. Neurology 2004;63(7): 1168–74.
2. Renner JA, Burns JM, Hou CE, et al. Progressive posterior cortical dysfunction: a clinicopathologic series. Neurology 2004;63(7):1175–80.
3. Josephs KA, Whitwell JL, Boeve BF, et al. Visual hallucinations in posterior cortical atrophy. Arch Neurol 2006;63(10):1427–32.
4. Victoroff J, Ross GW, Benson DF, et al. Posterior cortical atrophy. Neuropathologic correlations. Arch Neurol 1994;51(3):269–74.
5. Snowden JS, Stopford CL, Julien CL, et al. Cognitive phenotypes in Alzheimer's disease and genetic risk. Cortex 2007;43:835–45.
6. Mendez MF, Perryman KM. Posterior cortical atrophy: clinical characteristics and differences compared to Alzheimer's disease. Dement Geriatr Cogn Disord 2002; 14(1):33–40.
7. McMonagle P, Deering F, Berliner Y, et al. The cognitive profile of posterior cortical atrophy. Neurology 2006;66(3):331–8.
8. Charles RF, Hillis AE. Posterior cortical atrophy: clinical presentation and cognitive deficits compared to Alzheimer's disease. Behav Neurol 2005;16(1):15–23.
9. Howard R, Ballard C, O'Brien J, et al. Guidelines for the management of agitation in dementia. Int J Geriatr Psychiatry 2001;16(7):714–7.
10. McKeith IG, Dickson DW, Lowe J, et al. Diagnosis and management of dementia with Lewy bodies: third report of the DLB Consortium. Neurology 2005;65(12): 1863–72.
11. Kao AW, Racine CA, Quitania LC, et al. Cognitive and neuropsychiatric profile of the synucleinopathies: Parkinson disease, dementia with Lewy bodies, and multiple system atrophy. Alzheimer Dis Assoc Disord 2009;23(4):365–70.

12. Van Vliet D, de Vugt ME, Aalten P, et al. Prevalence of neuropsychiatric symptoms in young-onset compared to late-onset Alzheimer's disease - part 1: findings of the two-year longitudinal NeedYD-study. Dement Geriatr Cogn Disord 2012; 34(5–6):319–27.

13. Geda YE, Schneider LS, Gitlin LN, et al. Neuropsychiatric symptoms in Alzheimer's disease: past progress and anticipation of the future. Alzheimers Dement 2013;9(5):602–8.

14. Lyketsos CG, Carrillo MC, Ryan JM, et al. Neuropsychiatric symptoms in Alzheimer's disease. Alzheimers Dement 2011;7(5):532–9.

15. Lawlor A, Ryan M, Schmeidler J, et al. Clinical symptoms associated with age at onset in Alzheimer's disease. Am J Psychiatry 1994;151:1646–9.

16. Toyota Y, Ikeda M, Shinagawa S, et al. Comparison of behavioral and psychological symptoms in early-onset and late-onset Alzheimer's disease. Int J Geriatr Psychiatry 2007;22(9):896–901.

17. Rubin EH, Kinscherf DA, Morris JC. Psychopathology in younger versus older persons with very mild and mild dementia of the Alzheimer type. Am J Psychiatry 1993;150:639–42.

18. Isella V, Villa G, Mapelli C, et al. The neuropsychiatric profile of posterior cortical atrophy. J Geriatr Psychiatry Neurol 2014. [Epub ahead of print].

19. Aalten P, Verhey FR, Boziki M, et al. Consistency of neuropsychiatric syndromes across dementias: results from the European Alzheimer disease consortium. Dement Geriatr Cogn Disord 2008;25(1):1–8.

20. Steinberg M, Shao H, Zandi P, et al. Point and 5-year period prevalence of neuropsychiatric symptoms in dementia: the cache county study. Int J Geriatr Psychiatry 2008;23(2):170–7.

21. Shakespeare TJ, Yong KX, Foxe D, et al. Pronounced impairment of everyday skills and self-care in posterior cortical atrophy. J Alzheimers Dis 2015;43(2): 381–4.

22. Stella F, Radanovic M, Aprahamian I, et al. Neurobiological correlates of apathy in Alzheimer's disease and mild cognitive impairment: a critical review. J Alzheimers Dis 2014;39(3):633–48.

23. Theleritis C, Politis A, Siarkos K, et al. A review of neuroimaging findings of apathy in Alzheimer's disease. Int Psychogeriatr 2014;26(2):195–207.

24. D'Onofrio G, Sancarlo D, Panza F, et al. Neuropsychiatric symptoms and functional status in Alzheimer's disease and vascular dementia patients. Curr Alzheimer Res 2012;9(6):759–71.

25. Zhang M, Wang H, Li T, et al. Prevalence of neuropsychiatric symptoms across the declining memory continuum: an observational study in a memory clinic setting. Dement Geriatr Cogn Dis Extra 2012;2:200–8.

26. Del Prete M, Spaccavento S, Craca A, et al. Neuropsychiatric symptoms and the APOE genotype in Alzheimer's disease. Neurol Sci 2009;30(5):367–73.

27. Wolf RC, Schönfeldt-Lecuona C. Depressive symptoms as first manifestation of posterior cortical atrophy. Am J Psychiatry 2006;163(5):939–40.

28. Ownby RL, Crocco E, Acevedo A, et al. Depression and risk for Alzheimer disease: systematic review, meta-analysis, and metaregression analysis. Arch Gen Psychiatry 2006;63(5):530–8.

29. Aznar S, Knudsen GM. Depression and Alzheimer's disease: is stress the initiating factor in a common neuropathological cascade? J Alzheimers Dis 2011; 23(2):177–93.

30. Kessing LV. Depression and the risk for dementia. Curr Opin Psychiatry 2012; 25(6):457–61.

31. Alexopoulos GS, Kiosses DN, Choi SJ, et al. Frontal white matter microstructure and treatment response of late-life depression: a preliminary study. Am J Psychiatry 2002;159:1929–32.

32. Furuya H, Ikezoe K, Ohyagi Y, et al. A case of progressive posterior cortical atrophy (PCA) with vivid hallucination: are some ghost tales vivid hallucinations in normal people? J Neurol Neurosurg Psychiatry 2006;77(3):424–5.

33. Ballard C, Aarsland D, Francis P, et al. Neuropsychiatric symptoms in patients with dementias associated with cortical Lewy bodies: pathophysiology, clinical features, and pharmacological management. Drugs Aging 2013;30(8):603–11.

34. Yoshida T, Yuki N, Nakagawa M. Complex visual hallucination and mirror sign in posterior cortical atrophy. Acta Psychiatr Scand 2006;114(1):62–5.

35. Videaud H, Torny F, Cartz-Piver L, et al. Impact of drug-free care in posterior cortical atrophy: preliminary experience with a psycho-educative program. Rev Neurol (Paris) 2012;168:861–7.

36. Orgeta V, Qazi A, Ae S, et al. Psychological treatments for depression and anxiety in dementia and mild cognitive impairment. Cochrane Database Syst Rev 2014;(1):1–3.

37. Selwood A, Johnston K, Katona C, et al. Systematic review of the effect of psychological interventions on family caregivers of people with dementia. J Affect Disord 2007;101(1–3):75–89.

38. Clemerson G, Walsh S, Isaac C. Towards living well with young onset dementia: an exploration of coping from the perspective of those diagnosed. Dementia 2013;13(4):451–66.

39. Armari E, Jarmolowicz A, Panegyres PK. The needs of patients with early onset dementia. Am J Alzheimers Dis Other Demen 2013;28(1):42–6.

40. Gorno-Tempini ML, Hillis AE, Weintraub S, et al. Classification of primary progressive aphasia and its variants. Neurology 2011;76:1006–14.

41. Reder P, Fredman G. The relationship to help: interacting beliefs about the treatment process. Clin Child Psychol Psychiatry 1996;1(3):457–67.

42. Freyne A, Kidd N, Coen R, et al. Burden in carers of dementia patients. Higher levels in carers of younger sufferers. Int J Geriatr Psychiatry 1999;14:784–8.

43. Chu H, Yang CY, Liao YH, et al. The effects of a support group on dementia caregivers' burden and depression. J Aging Health 2011;23(2):228–41.

Rapidly Progressive Young-Onset Dementias
Neuropsychiatric Aspects

Rajeet Shrestha, MD[a,b], Timothy Wuerz, DO[a],
Brian S. Appleby, MD[a,b,c],*

KEYWORDS

- Rapidly progressive dementia • Young onset dementia • Early onset dementia
- Presenile dementia • Neuropsychiatry • Prion disease • Creutzfeldt–Jakob disease
- Neuropsychiatric symptoms

KEY POINTS

- Rapidly progressive dementia (RPD) is roughly defined as progression to dementia or death within 2 years.
- Many RPDs demonstrate neuropsychiatric symptoms, especially at initial presentation.
- The differential diagnosis for RPD in younger patients is broad. Diagnostic workup includes blood work, brain MRI, electroencephalogram (EEG), lumbar puncture, and body CT.
- Creutzfeldt–Jakob disease is diagnosed clinically by assessing a clinical syndrome as well as the use of EEG, cerebrospinal fluid 14-3-3 proteins, and brain MRI findings.
- Clinical management should employ nonpharmacologic interventions first, followed by pharmacologic treatments if necessary. Neuropsychiatric symptoms should be reassessed frequently and medications adjusted as necessary.

INTRODUCTION

Rapidly progressive dementias (RPDs) are a unique and important population of patients of which psychiatrists should be aware. Many RPDs occur in younger

Support for this article was provided in part by a University Hospitals Spitz Award and the Stivison Fund for CJD Research.

a Department of Neurology, Case Western Reserve University School of Medicine & University Hospitals, 3619 Park East Drive, Suite 211, Beachwood, OH 44122, USA; b Department of Psychiatry, Case Western Reserve University School of Medicine & University Hospitals, 3619 Park East Drive, Suite 211, Beachwood, OH 44122, USA; c Department of Pathology, Case Western Reserve University School of Medicine & University Hospitals, 3619 Park East Drive, Suite 211, Beachwood, OH 44122, USA
* Corresponding author. 3619 Park East Drive, Suite 206, Beachwood, OH 44122.
E-mail address: bsa35@case.edu

Psychiatr Clin N Am 38 (2015) 221–232
http://dx.doi.org/10.1016/j.psc.2015.01.001
0193-953X/15/$ – see front matter © 2015 Elsevier Inc. All rights reserved.

Abbreviations	
AD	Alzheimer's disease
APOE	Apolipoprotein E gene
CJD	Creutzfeldt–Jakob disease
CSF	Cerebrospinal fluid
EEG	Electroencephalogram
FTLD	Frontotemporal lobar degeneration
PRNP	Prion protein gene
PrPc	Native cellular prion protein
PrPSc	Pathologic scrapie prion protein
rpAD	Rapidly progressive Alzheimer's disease
RPD	Rapidly progressive dementia
RT-QuIC	Real-time quaking-induced conversion
sCJD	Sporadic Creutzfeldt–Jakob disease
vCJD	Variant Creutzfeldt–Jakob disease
YOAD	Young-onset Alzheimer's disease
YOD	Young-onset dementia

patients, in which sense they overlap with young-onset dementias (YODs). Both groups frequently exhibit a clinical presentation in which neuropsychiatric symptoms are prominent. For the purposes of this discussion, YOD refers to cases in which signs and symptoms of dementia start to occur before the age of 65. RPD is roughly defined as cases in which severe dementia or death occur within 2 years of symptom onset. This article discusses the differential diagnosis, workup, and management of this population with emphasis on certain patient groups.

DIFFERENTIAL DIAGNOSIS

The differential diagnosis of RPD is extensive and includes neurodegenerative, inflammatory/autoimmune, infectious, toxic–metabolic, and neoplastic causes, among others (**Box 1**). The most common etiology for RPD is neurodegenerative diseases, which do not have disease-modifying treatments. Prion diseases are usually high in the differential diagnosis when evaluating a patient with RPD, but other etiologies must be considered. Other neurodegenerative diseases typically have a slow progression, but they can sometimes be rapidly progressive.

Non-neurodegenerative causes of RPD can be treated potentially and their course halted or reversed to varying degrees. If undiagnosed or untreated, a number of these conditions may progress rapidly and be fatal. Therefore, it is paramount to investigate comprehensively and expeditiously any presentation of a rapid deterioration in cognitive, behavioral, and motor functioning. Among nondegenerative etiologies, autoimmune diseases form a major diagnostic group that includes encephalopathies associated with antineuronal antibodies, steroid responsive encephalopathy with associated autoimmune thyroiditis, central nervous system lupus, multiple sclerosis, and others. A number of infectious diseases can also affect the brain and can be difficult to diagnose clinically if there are no other obvious clinical signs of infection. Various vitamin deficiencies, endocrine and metabolic disorders, and toxicities should also be considered in cases of RPD. Finally, primary central nervous system neoplastic causes should be ruled out.[1]

EPIDEMIOLOGY

The epidemiologic characteristics of RPD are highly variable because of the diverse etiologic conditions that can lead to them. Individuals with AD and dementia with

Box 1
Differential diagnoses of rapidly progressive dementia

Underlying Etiology	Examples
Neurodegenerative	Alzheimer disease
	Frontotemporal lobar degeneration
	Dementia with Lewy bodies
	Corticobasal degeneration
	Progressive supranuclear palsy
	Prion disease
Inflammatory/autoimmune	Antineuronal antibody mediated (eg, VGKC complex, NMDAR, anti-Hu, anti-Ma)
	Steroid responsive encephalopathy associated with autoimmune thyroiditis
	CNS lupus
	Multiple sclerosis
	Sarcoidosis
	Behçet disease
	CNS vasculitis
Infectious	Prion disease
	Syphilis
	HIV dementia
	Meningitis
	Encephalitis (eg, herpes simplex virus)
	Progressive multifocal leukoencephalopathy (JC virus)
	CNS fungal infections
	Whipple's disease
Toxic–metabolic	Alcohol
	Heavy metals (eg, mercury, arsenic)
	Carbon monoxide
	Lithium toxicity
	Vitamin deficiencies (B_1, B_{12}, niacin)
	Hepatic encephalopathy
	Uremia
	Electrolyte disturbance
Neoplastic	Primary CNS lymphoma
	Metastases to CNS
	Paraneoplastic syndromes
Vascular	Stroke
	Binswanger disease
Endocrine	Hypo- and hyper- thyroid and parathyroid, and adrenal states

Abbreviations: CNS, central nervous system; HIV, human immunodeficiency virus; JC virus, John Cunningham virus; NMDAR, *N*-methyl-D-aspartate receptor; VGKC, voltage-gated potassium channel.

Lewy bodies tend to have older mean ages at disease onset, whereas FTLD often presents in mid-to-late life. Depending on the etiology, the mean age at onset of prion disease varies from very young (variant Creutzfeldt–Jakob disease [CJD]) to mid/late life (genetic and sporadic CJD).[2] The demographic distribution of the paraneoplastic encephalopathies show a wide range depending on the antibodies involved—for instance, there is a female predominance in anti–*N*-methyl-D-aspartate receptor encephalitis and the median age at onset is 19 years whereas, the median age at onset for encephalitis associated with voltage-gated potassium channel antibodies is 60 years. In the case of infectious causes, the at-risk population as well as geographic prevalence of the particular infection influences the epidemiologic characteristics.

Similarly, toxic and metabolic causes are seen more commonly in populations at risk for those particular conditions. Vascular dementias generally occur in patients who are over 50 years of age and in those with risk factors for vascular disease.[3]

EVALUATION OF RAPIDLY PROGRESSIVE DEMENTIA

Any evaluation of a rapid progression of cognitive, behavioral, and motor functioning must begin with a comprehensive history, including details about the onset, course, and progression of symptoms, with particular attention to their order of appearance (**Fig. 1**). The domains of cognition, behavior, motor and sensory functions involved, the time evolution of symptoms, and the ensuing patterns are important to note. Any change in personality and social behaviors, including disinhibition or apathy, should be assessed specifically. Change in dietary preferences, if present, may also be significant. Any factors that alleviate or exacerbate symptoms should be enquired about. A thorough review of neuropsychiatric as well as physical symptoms should be conducted. Medical and surgical history, current medication regimen, and any changes in medications especially that coincide with onset or change in the nature and/or severity of symptoms should be assessed carefully. Personal history should include extent and patterns of substance use, occupational history including exposure to any toxins, and premorbid level of functioning. Finally, a family history of neurodegenerative dementia, movement disorders, autoimmune disorders, psychiatric disorders, and suicide should be sought.[4]

A thorough neuropsychiatric examination should be conducted after the history has been obtained. Neurologic examination should include evaluation of the cranial

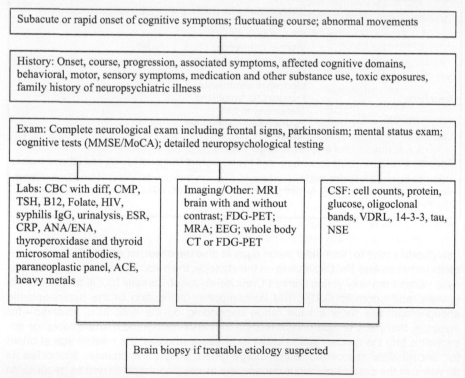

Fig. 1. Flowchart of proposed workup for rapidly progressive dementia.

nerves, motor abilities, abnormal movements and muscular tone, cerebellar functioning, gait, and frontal release signs. A complete mental status examination should include evaluation of mood, affect, anxiety levels, obsessions, compulsions, perceptual disturbances, hallucinations, delusions, agitation/aggression, thought processes, and suicidal thoughts or passive death wishes. Office testing of major cognitive domains, including memory, language, visuospatial and executive functioning should be conducted; this testing can be done through standardized screening tests such as the Montreal Cognitive Assessment[5] or Mini-Mental Status Examination.[6] Further evaluation of cognitive functioning can be done through more detailed office testing or comprehensive neuropsychological testing performed by a neuropsychologist.

Laboratory testing for evaluation of RPD should start with basic tests for reversible dementias. Basic diagnostics include complete blood count with differential, serum chemistry, vitamin B_{12}, folic acid, thyroid stimulating hormone, urinalysis, and tests for human immunodeficiency virus and syphilis. The broader differential diagnosis involved in RPD compared with other forms of dementia warrants more extensive laboratory investigations. Inflammatory makers, such as erythrocyte sedimentation rate and C-reactive protein, autoantibodies for connective tissue disorders such as antinuclear antibodies and extractable nuclear antibodies, as well as a paraneoplastic antibody panel, should also be ordered. Serum angiotensin-converting enzyme levels should be tested if sarcoidosis is suspected owing to cranial nerve involvement, pulmonary symptoms, and/or the presence of enhancing lesions on brain MRI after administration of gadolinium. In contrast with routine evaluation and management of dementias with features typical of common neurodegenerative conditions where a spinal tap is usually not necessary, cerebrospinal fluid (CSF) analysis for detecting the presence of inflammatory or infectious disease markers may be of diagnostic value in case of RPD. This analysis should include CSF biomarkers for CJD including 14-3-3, tau, and neuron-specific enolase.

Brain imaging is a vital part of the diagnostic workup for all patients with cognitive deterioration. Brain MRI (with and without gadolinium) is recommended for all patients with RPD. MR angiography should be considered if there is concern for a vascular etiology for the dementia because of sudden symptom onset or stepwise progression of symptoms. Electroencephalogram (EEG), although nonspecific, can be a useful diagnostic tool to assess for epileptiform activity or periodic sharp wave complexes, which are suggestive of prion disease. Brain fluorodeoxyglucose positron emission tomography can be used to distinguish FTLD from posterior pathologic processes (eg, AD). Although rarely used, brain biopsy can be considered if other investigations are uninformative diagnostically and there is concern of a treatable cause of RPD that a biopsy would help to inform. An example of an appropriate use of brain biopsy is collecting tissue from a focal gadolinium-enhancing lesion observed on brain MRI that is likely neoplastic in origin. In this instance, brain biopsy informs diagnosis, prognosis, and potential treatment options. In the absence of an overt etiology, a chest/abdomen/pelvis CT with contrast or body fluorodeoxyglucose positron emission tomography is performed to rule out neoplastic and paraneoplastic processes, even if paraneoplastic antibody panels are negative.

SPECIFIC ETIOLOGIES OF RAPIDLY PROGRESSIVE DEMENTIA
Prion Disease

Prion diseases are rapidly progressive neurodegenerative diseases caused by an abnormal conformation of the native cellular prion protein (PrP^c). According to the "protein-only" hypothesis, the pathologic scrapie prion protein (PrPSc) is both necessary and sufficient to produce prion disease.[7] Prion diseases are transmissible in specific circumstances and are thus sometimes referred to as transmissible spongiform encephalopathy. Through template-directed misfolding, PrPSc converts PrP^c into further PrPSc in an autocatalytic cycle. Prion diseases are characterized neuropathologically by spongiform changes, astrocytosis, and neuronal loss.[8] The estimated incidence of human prion disease is 1 to 2 new cases per million people per year.

Human prion diseases have 3 possible etiologies: sporadic, genetic, and acquired. The majority of prion diseases (85%) are thought to be of sporadic etiology owing to a posttranslational modification of PrP^c into PrPSc.[8] Approximately 10% to 15% of prion diseases are owing to genetic mutations of the prion protein gene (PRNP) that are named according to their clinical and neuropathologic phenotype. Most genetic prion diseases are termed genetic CJD because of its resemblance to sporadic CJD (sCJD) and are caused most frequently by autosomal-dominant point mutations.[9] Another genetic prion disease is Gerstmann–Sträussler–Scheinker syndrome caused by several different PRNP mutations and characterized by longer illness durations (several years as opposed to several months in most cases of CJD), early and prominent cerebellar symptoms (eg, gait ataxia, vertigo, nystagmus, incoordination), and kuru plaques in the cerebellum. Fatal familial insomnia is caused by a mutation at codon 178 paired with methionine at codon 129 on the mutated PRNP allele, resulting in profound thalamic degeneration with resulting autonomic dysfunction and sleep disturbances manifest as labile blood pressure and pulse, pyrexia, and loss of sleep architecture on EEG, usually resulting in daytime somnolence and parasomnias. The remainder of prion diseases (<1%) are acquired.[10] Prion disease can be acquired via ritualistic endocannabalism (ie, kuru),[11] through specific medical procedures (iatrogenic CJD),[12] or through the ingestion of food contaminated with bovine spongiform encephalopathy (variant CJD).[13]

Demographically, sCJD may be considered the prototypic rapidly progressive YOD. The mean age at onset of sCJD is approximately 61 years of age and the mean survival time from symptom onset until death is under 1 year.[14] Men and women seem to be affected equally and there are some variations in age of onset and survival time depending on race/ethnicity.[15] For example, non-Hispanic whites tend to have an older age at disease onset compared with other racial and ethnic groups. Although the only way to definitely diagnose sCJD is via autopsy, antemortem diagnosis can be reliably achieved. Diagnostic criteria involve the synthesis of clinical symptoms and diagnostic test results (Box 2).[16] Further CSF tests can be helpful. For example, sCJD is unique in its characteristic highly elevated CSF tau levels (>1150 pg/mL), which is a fairly specific diagnostic test.[17] Recently developed, real-time quaking-induced conversion (RT-QuIC) is able to detect PrPSc within the CSF using a modified approach of protein misfolding cyclic amplification, yielding a specificity of 99% to 100% across most performing laboratories.[18,19] Current research is also investigating using RT-QuIC testing on olfactory epithelium via noninvasive nasal brushings.[20]

Psychiatrists should be knowledgeable about prion diseases because of the multiple psychiatric symptoms that may lead to a psychiatric evaluation. Approximately 16% of prion disease cases are initially misdiagnosed as a primary psychiatric illness.[21] Across all types of prion disease, cognitive impairment is the most common neuropsychiatric symptom, followed by behavior/personality changes (~20%), affective illness (~14%), and psychosis/agitation (~11%).[14] Younger sCJD patients (<50 years of age) tend to present more often with affective illness (~28% vs ~1%), which may partly describe why variant CJD (vCJD) patients often present with psychiatric symptoms (see below). In one study,[22] approximately 15% of patients

---

Box 2
Diagnostic criteria for probable sporadic Creutzfeldt–Jakob disease

Clinical Symptoms: Must have dementia and at least 2 of the following:

A. Visual or cerebellar symptoms

B. Pyramidal or extrapyramidal symptoms

C. Myoclonus

D. Akinetic mutism

Diagnostic tests: Must have at least 1 of the following:

A. Periodic sharp wave complexes on electroencephalogram

B. Cerebrospinal fluid 14-3-3 protein and duration less than 2 years

C. Hyperintensity on brain MRI DWI/FLAIR sequences in the caudate and putamen, and/or 2 or more cortical areas (temporal, parietal, occipital)

Abbreviations: DWI, diffusion weighted imaging; FLAIR, fluid attenuated inversion recovery.

---

with sCJD presented solely with affective symptoms. These affective phenotype cases tended to be younger, had a prolonged time to clinical presentation and diagnostic testing, had survival times of greater than 6 months typically, and had a high rate of positive CSF 14-3-3 protein.[22]

vCJD is characterized by its prominent early neuropsychiatric symptoms in young patients, factors that were essential for its initial detection in the United Kingdom.[13] Neuropsychiatric presentations are common and are often the only presenting symptom.[23] Common psychiatric symptoms in vCJD include mood lability, anxiety, apathy, aggression, insomnia, depression, delusions, and hallucinations. Although EEG and CSF 14-3-3 protein are often unrevealing, the brain MRI of patients with vCJD often demonstrate the pulvinar sign (sensitivity of 78% and specificity of 100%), which is hyperintensity of the pulvinar nucleus of the thalamus.[24] This brain MRI finding usually occurs in isolation and without other neuroimaging findings typically seen in sCJD. Given the frequent psychiatric presentations in all forms of prion disease, diagnosis of prion disease should be entertained in younger individuals with these symptoms who rapidly develop other neurologic symptoms. Treatment of psychiatric symptoms in prion disease is symptom based and supportive in nature.[25]

Alzheimer Disease

AD is the most common neurodegenerative cause of dementia across all age groups, and comprises about half of YODs (<65 years of age). Genetic mutations of 3 genes (*Presenilin 1 gene*, *Presenilin 2 gene*, *Amyloid precursor protein gene*) are known to cause approximately 2% of AD cases.[26] Inheritance is autosomal dominant, with near-complete penetrance and clinical presentation of symptoms usually occurs before 60 years of age. However, most cases of young-onset AD (YOAD) are not owing to a genetic mutation, but are sporadic in etiology. Similar to sCJD, YOAD seems to be more prevalent in certain minority populations (Native American Indian, Alaskan, Hawaiian, and Hispanics).[27] Common risk factors for late-onset AD, such as *Apolipoprotein E4 gene* (*APOE4*) alleles, hypertension, stroke, and atrial fibrillation, are less common in YOAD.[27,28] Approximately one-third of those with YOAD have an atypical, nonamnestic presentation that often leads to an incorrect initial diagnosis.[29] YOAD patients also have more anxiety and depressive symptoms compared with late-onset AD patients,[27,30] possibly owing to higher awareness of their disabilities.[31] Apathy is another common neuropsychiatric symptom observed in YOAD.[32]

A rare subset of AD is rapidly progressive AD (rpAD). Although the criteria for what constitutes rpAD is still up for debate, Schmidt and colleagues[33] propose a decrement of 6 or more points per year on the Mini-Mental State Examination. Depending on the criteria used to define rpAD, approximately 10% to 30% of all AD cases may be considered rapidly progressive. Mean age at disease onset is unclear, although it seems to be roughly equivalent to that seen in non-rpAD cases.[33,34] Average survival time is approximately 2 to 3 years and focal neurologic signs (especially extrapyramidal symptoms) occur early in the disease course. Other frequent neurologic symptoms include myoclonus (75%) and disturbed gait (66%).[35] CSF study results also can resemble that seen in prion disease, with elevated total tau levels and positive 14-3-3 proteins. However, CSF p-tau levels are also elevated in rpAD, whereas they are not in prion disease. Interestingly, there is an underrepresentation of *APOE4* alleles in rpAD than what would be normally expected in AD.[33,36] rpAD can mimic symptoms of prion disease and is often misdiagnosed as such. In fact, 66% of untreatable illnesses misdiagnosed as prion disease were found to be AD at autopsy in a National Prion Disease Pathology Surveillance Center series.[37]

MANAGEMENT

General management considerations can be applied to the progressive stages of RPD (mild, moderate, and severe/end stage; **Table 1**). Nonpharmacologic strategies

Table 1
Symptomatic treatment recommendations

Symptom	Suggested Treatment
Depression/anxiety	Nonpharmacologic: counseling; art, music, and aroma therapy Pharmacologic: SSRIs; mirtazapine; trazodone; benzodiazepines
Psychosis/agitation	Nonpharmacologic: art, music, and aroma therapy; ensuring basic biological needs are being met; frequent toileting Pharmacologic: SSRIs; trazodone; low potency neuroleptics (eg, quetiapine); valproic acid; benzodiazepines
Myoclonus/hyperstartle	Nonpharmacologic: minimize stimulation through limited number of visits and visitors; remove telephone from patient room; tape over doorbell; move patient away from the nursing station owing to increased stimulation with change of shift Pharmacologic: long-acting benzodiazepines (eg, diazepam); anticonvulsants (eg, valproic acid)
Seizures	Anticonvulsants
Dystonia/contractures	Nonpharmacologic: passive movement exercises Pharmacologic: long-acting benzodiazepines; Botulinum toxin injections
Sleep disorders	Nonpharmacologic: good sleep hygiene; routine sleep schedule Pharmacologic: melatonin; trazodone; benzodiazepines (REM sleep behavior disorder); dopamine agonists (restless legs syndrome)
Constipation	Bowel regimen (eg, Dulcolax)
Dysphagia/rumination	Thickener; cueing; different textured food at varying temperatures

Abbreviations: REM, rapid eye movement; SSRI, selective serotonin reuptake inhibitor.

should be implemented first and include art/music therapy, aroma and natural oils therapy, and supportive counseling. Environmental changes are important in terms of adding handicap features to the bathroom, removing floor obstacles to avoid tripping, limiting or avoiding high-stimulating television programs, and setting up reminder aids like clocks and calendars. Mild to moderate stages benefit from both drug and nondrug approaches. Pharmacologically, selective serotonin reuptake inhibitor trials can be started to target neuropsychiatric symptoms like anxiety, depression, or behavioral disturbances. At times, psychotic and behavioral symptoms may become severe and require an atypical antipsychotic like quetiapine, which has the lowest risk of extrapyramidal side effects. However, caution must be taken with neuroleptics in cases of dementia with Lewy bodies owing to the greater risk for neuroleptic malignant syndrome and delirium. Cholinesterase inhibitors can be useful in dementia with Lewy bodies for perceptual disturbances and should be tried first.[38] If not helpful, very judicious use of quetiapine may be attempted (ie, start at 12.5 mg/d). Benzodiazepines, like clonazepam, can be helpful with management of episodic anxiety, rapid eye movement sleep behavior disorder, and myoclonus. However, use of benzodiazepines requires close monitoring for paradoxic disinhibition that can occur in some cases. Melatonin can be used to assist with the sleep–wake cycle. Social work consultation can also be helpful early in the disease course. Of note, many etiologies of RPD are on the Social Security Disability Insurance Compassionate Allowances List, which waives the usual 2-year waiting period between disability approval and its subsequent payments (http://www.ssa.gov/compassionateallowances/conditions.htm).

End-stage dementia is a difficult time emotionally and physically for both patients and their families. A hospice referral is highly recommended and the following can help to steer clinicians toward when it is appropriate to consult palliative care. In general, hospice requires several eligibility criteria before admission (**Box 3**).[39] In addition to the palliative care elements of hospice, they also provide several other important ancillary services, including support structure, readily available resources, nursing

---

Box 3
Hospice eligibility criteria for people with dementia

All of the following:

- Unable to ambulate without assistance
- Unable to dress without assistance
- Unable to bath without assistance
- Urinary or fecal incontinence intermittent or constant
- No consistent meaningful verbal communication; speech is limited to 6 or fewer intelligible words or only stereotypical phrases

One of the following within the past 12 months:

- Aspiration pneumonia
- Pyelonephritis or upper urinary tract infection
- Septicemia
- Decubitus ulcers, multiple, stages 3–4
- Fever, recurrent after antibiotics
- Inability to maintain sufficient fluid and calorie intake with 10% weight loss during the previous 6 months or serum albumin less than 2.5 gm/dL

visits, bereavement counseling, medical equipment supplies, dietary counseling, and spiritual counseling.

Overall, each stage of a RPD requires close clinical follow-up. Patients may require monthly visits during the mild stage of illness and weekly follow-ups with possible home visits during the end stages. The physician's role once hospice has been established varies and depends largely on individual preferences and comfort with palliative care. Nursing visits are provided as part of hospice care and the physician may choose to be the attending hospice doctor on record or continue as a consultant. Reimbursement rules change when a patient is in hospice care and the hospice social worker or nurse can usually guide the provider in how to bill for his or her services. During these visits, reassessment of treatment, including medication adjustment is warranted, because the progression is rapid. In addition, supportive agencies like the CJD Foundation (www.cjdfoundation.org), Alzheimer's Association (www.alz.org), and The Association for Frontotemporal Degeneration (www.theaftd.org) are very helpful for accessing resources and education.

SUMMARY

RPD commonly occurs in younger patients and frequently demonstrates neuropsychiatric phenomena. The clinical phenomenology, varied differential diagnoses and subsequent management options require that psychiatrists have some familiarity with this patient population. Achieving the correct diagnosis by investigating all possible causes through the workup process described herein is essential owing to possible treatable causes of RPD. Education, communication, and symptom management are the mainstays of treatment for RPD and aptly suited for individuals with training in psychiatry.

REFERENCES

1. Geschwind MD, Haman A, Miller BL. Rapidly progressive dementia. Neurol Clin 2007;25(3):783–807.
2. Appleby B. Prion diseases. In: Abou-Saleh M, Katona C, Kumar A, editors. Principles and practice of geriatric psychiatry. 3rd edition. New York: John Wiley & Sons, Inc; 2011. p. 372–7.
3. Paterson RW, Torres-Chae CC, Kuo AL, et al. Differential diagnosis of Jakob-Creutzfeldt disease. Arch Neurol 2012;69(12):1578–82.
4. Rosenbloom MH, Atri A. The evaluation of rapidly progressive dementia. Neurologist 2011;17(2):67–74.
5. Nasreddine ZS, Phillips NA, Bédirian V, et al. The Montreal Cognitive Assessment, MoCA: a brief screening tool for mild cognitive impairment. J Am Geriatr Soc 2005;53(4):695–9.
6. Folstein MF, Folstein SE, McHugh PR. "Mini-mental state." A practical method for grading the cognitive state of patients for the clinician. J Psychiatr Res 1975; 12(3):189–98.
7. Prusiner SB. Novel proteinaceous infectious particles cause scrapie. Science 1982;216(4542):136–44.
8. World Health Organization (WHO). Global surveillance, diagnosis and therapy of human transmissible spongiform encephalopathies: report of a WHO consultation. Geneva (Switzerland): World Health Organization; 1998.
9. Kong Q. Inherited prion diseases. In: Prusiner SB, editor. Prion biology and diseases. 2nd edition. Cold Spring Harbor (NY): Cold Spring Harbor Laboratory Press; 2004. p. 673–775.

10. Will R. Acquired prion disease: iatrogenic CJD, variant CJD, kuru. Br Med Bull 2003;66(1):255–65.
11. Gajdusek D, Zigas V. Degenerative disease of the central nervous system in New Guinea; the endemic occurrence of kuru in the native population. N Engl J Med 1957;257(20):974–8.
12. Brown P, Brandel J-P, Sato T, et al. Iatrogenic Creutzfeldt-Jakob disease, final assessment. Emerg Infect Dis 2012;18(6):901–7.
13. Will R, Ironside J. A new variant of Creutzfeldt-Jakob disease in the UK. Lancet 1996;347(9006):921.
14. Appleby BS, Appleby KK, Rabins PV. Does the presentation of Creutzfeldt-Jakob disease vary by age or presumed etiology? A meta-analysis of the past 10 years. J Neuropsychiatry Clin Neurosci 2007;19(4):428–35.
15. Appleby BS, Rincon-Beardsley TD, Appleby KK, et al. Racial and ethnic differences in individuals with sporadic Creutzfeldt-Jakob disease in the United States of America. PLos One 2012;7(6):e38884.
16. Zerr I, Kallenberg K, Summers DM, et al. Updated clinical diagnostic criteria for sporadic Creutzfeldt Jakob disease. Brain 2009;132(Pt 10):2659–68.
17. Hamlin C, Puoti G, Berri S, et al. A comparison of tau and 14-3-3 protein in the diagnosis of Creutzfeldt-Jakob disease. Neurology 2012;79(6):547–52.
18. Atarashi R, Satoh K, Sano K, et al. Ultrasensitive human prion detection in cerebrospinal fluid by real-time quaking-induced conversion. Nat Med 2011;17(2):175–8.
19. McGuire LI, Peden AH, Orrù CD, et al. Real time quaking-induced conversion analysis of cerebrospinal fluid in sporadic Creutzfeldt-Jakob disease. Ann Neurol 2012;72(2):278–85.
20. Orrù CD, Bongianni M, Tonoli G, et al. A test for Creutzfeldt-Jakob disease using nasal brushings. N Engl J Med 2014;371(6):519–29.
21. Appleby BS, Rincon-Beardsley TD, Appleby KK, et al. Initial diagnoses of patients ultimately diagnosed with prion disease. J Alzheimers Dis 2014;42(3):833–9.
22. Appleby BS, Appleby KK, Crain BJ, et al. Characteristics of established and proposed sporadic Creutzfeldt-Jakob disease variants. Arch Neurol 2009;66(2):208–15.
23. Zeidler M, Johnstone EC, Bamber RW, et al. New variant Creutzfeldt-Jakob disease: psychiatric features. Lancet 1997;350(9082):908–10.
24. Zeidler M, Sellar RJ, Collie DA, et al. The pulvinar sign on magnetic resonance imaging in variant Creutzfeldt-Jakob disease. Lancet 2000;355(9213):1412–8.
25. Thompson A, MacKay A, Rudge P, et al. Behavioral and psychiatric symptoms in prion disease. Am J Psychiatry 2014;171(3):265–74.
26. Greicius MD, Geschwind MD, Miller BL. Presenile dementia syndromes: an update on taxonomy and diagnosis. J Neurol Neurosurg Psychiatry 2002;72(6):691–700.
27. Panegyres PK, Chen HY, Coalition against Major Diseases (CAMD). Early-onset Alzheimer's disease: a global cross-sectional analysis. Eur J Neurol 2014;21(9):1149–54.
28. Panegyres PK, Chen HY. Differences between early and late onset Alzheimer's disease. Am J Neurodegener Dis 2013;2(4):300–6.
29. Balasa M, Gelpi E, Antonell A, et al. Clinical features and APOE genotype of pathologically proven early-onset Alzheimer disease. Neurology 2011;76(20):1720–5.
30. Kaiser NC, Liang LJ, Melrose RJ. Differences in anxiety among patients with early-versus late-onset Alzheimer's disease. J Neuropsychiatry Clin Neurosci 2014;26(1):73–80.

31. van Vliet D, de Vugt ME, Köhler S, et al. Awareness and its association with affective symptoms in young-onset and late-onset Alzheimer disease: a prospective study. Alzheimer Dis Assoc Disord 2013;27(3):265–71.
32. van Vliet D, de Vugt ME, Aalten P, et al. Prevalence of neuropsychiatric symptoms in young-onset compared to late-onset Alzheimer's disease - part 1: findings of the two-year longitudinal needYD-study. Dement Geriatr Cogn Disord 2012; 34(5–6):319–27.
33. Schmidt C, Wolff M, Weitz M, et al. Rapidly progressive Alzheimer disease. Arch Neurol 2011;68(9):1124–30.
34. Mann UM, Mohr E, Chase TN. Rapidly progressive Alzheimer's disease. Lancet 1989;2(8666):799.
35. Schmidt C, Redyk K, Meissner B, et al. Clinical features of rapidly progressive Alzheimer's disease. Dement Geriatr Cogn Disord 2010;29(4):371–8.
36. Schmidt C, Haïk S, Satoh K, et al. Rapidly progressive Alzheimer's disease: a multicenter update. J Alzheimers Dis 2012;30(4):751–6.
37. Chitravas N, Jung RS, Kofskey DM, et al. Treatable neurological disorders misdiagnosed as Creutzfeldt-Jakob disease. Ann Neurol 2011;70(3):437–44.
38. Racine CA. Dementia with Lewy bodies. In: Miller BL, Boeve BF, editors. The behavioral neurology of dementia. 1st edition. Cambridge (United Kingdom): Cambridge University Press; 2009. p. 7–26.
39. Storey CP. A Quick-Reference Guide to the Hospice and Palliative Care Training for Physicians: UNIPC Self-Study Program. American Academy of Hospice and Palliative Medicine; 2009.

Young-Onset Dementia Epidemiology Applied to Neuropsychiatry Practice

Bhargavi Devineni, MBBS[a], Chiadi U. Onyike, MD, MHS[b],*

KEYWORDS

- Young-onset dementia • Epidemiology • Risk factors • Differential diagnosis
- Screening

KEY POINTS

- Young-onset dementia (YOD) is an important clinical and epidemiologic problem that is often overshadowed in clinical and public consciousness.
- Neurodegenerative diseases are the leading cause of YOD. Alzheimer disease (AD) is most common, followed closely by frontotemporal dementia and vascular dementia.
- YOD may have nonamnesic, psychiatric, and neurologic presentations.
- An algorithmic approach to interpreting clinical data, based on defining syndromes, facilitates preliminary diagnosis and guides diagnostic testing.
- Screening for YOD in the psychiatric context is a rational process in which vigilance is combined with careful searches for red flags that signal a psychiatric state is neurodegenerative.

INTRODUCTION

Young-onset presentations of dementia are increasingly recognized as important causes of midlife morbidity and mortality. Young-onset dementia (YOD), typically defined as dementia arising before the age of 65, is also referred to as *early-onset dementia* (and in older times it was commonly known as presenile dementia). This age threshold, albeit socially determined and arbitrary, has proved useful for practice innovations and for research. It has, for example, provided a framework for distinguishing YODs from the more common late-life occurrences. This distinction serves important differences in etiology, phenotypes, handicaps, psychosocial difficulties

Disclosures: Dr Devineni has nothing to disclose. Dr Onyike is supported by the Johns Hopkins Alzheimer's Disease Research Center (National Institutes on Aging grant P50AG05146), the Jane Tanger Black Fund for Young-Onset Dementia Research, and the Robert Hall family.
[a] Geriatric Psychiatry Division, Department of Psychiatry, Zucker Hillside Hospital, 75-59 263rd Street, Glen Oaks, NY 11004, USA; [b] Department of Psychiatry and Behavioral Sciences, Johns Hopkins University School of Medicine, 600 North Wolfe Street, Meyer 279, Baltimore, MD 21287, USA
* Corresponding author.
E-mail address: conyike1@jhmi.edu

Psychiatr Clin N Am 38 (2015) 233–248
http://dx.doi.org/10.1016/j.psc.2015.02.003
0193-953X/15/$ – see front matter © 2015 Elsevier Inc. All rights reserved.

Abbreviations	
AD	Alzheimer disease
ALS	Amyotrophic lateral sclerosis
ARD	Alcohol-related dementia
CBD	Corticobasal degeneration
CJD	Creutzfeldt-Jakob disease
DLB	Dementia with Lewy bodies
FTD	Frontotemporal dementia
FTD-ALS	FTD with amyotrophic lateral sclerosis
HD	Huntington disease
PDD	Parkinson disease
PSP	Progressive supranuclear palsy
SD	Semantic dementia
TBI	Traumatic brain injury
VaD	Vascular dementia
YOD	Young-onset dementia

and, ultimately, clinical care. Whereas late-life dementias are, with the exception of those stemming from cerebrovascular disease, generally neurodegenerative, the YODs are more heterogeneous. It is the case that most YODs are neurodegenerative, but many cases arise from genetic, infectious, autoimmune, vascular, nutritional, and metabolic etiologies.

YOD is overshadowed in the clinical and public consciousness by the perception that dementia, which is more common in later life, is exclusively suffered by the elderly. Owing to this low public awareness, and physicians' lack of familiarity with the various conditions from which YOD arises, the diagnosis is frequently missed or late. For example, one study found an average time to diagnosis of 4.5 years, which was 1.6 years longer than for the late-onset group in that study.[1]

Knowledge among clinicians and the public of the clinical and demographic characteristics of YOD will facilitate recognition and accurate diagnosis and, thereby, prompt and effective care. Effective care includes treatment of the neuropsychiatric facets of these disorders and management of the psychosocial needs of the individuals and families. YOD frequently manifests neuropsychiatric phenomena alongside impairments of cognitive functions, often presenting with abnormalities of affect, temperament, judgment, dispositions and self-control, perception, ideation, and subsistence behaviors (feeding, elimination, sexual expression, and sleep). The psychosocial problems arising from these conditions include conflict, financial strain (as the patient may be a primary breadwinner or the caregiver of children), emotional stress on spouses (and other relatives) who provide care, work, and parenting and suffer social disconnection caused by distraction and isolation.[2] Children of individuals who suffer YODs also suffer adaptation-related stresses.[3,4] Thus, YOD is topical for psychiatry because of the phenotypes, the psychosocial dimensions of the suffering, and the skillset of the specialty. Psychiatrists, by virtue of their multidimensional training and professional orientation, have the tools to treat the illness, manage the problems, and direct the rehabilitation.

This report, like others in this issue, provides an introduction to aspects of YOD that are important for psychiatric practice. The clinical epidemiology of the neurodegenerative forms of YOD are discussed, including the pertinence to clinical work. The demographic and phenotypic attributes of YOD that form clues aiding the clinical recognition of the various etiologic types are discussed. Screening and measurement are also covered. The aim is to provide psychiatrists and other mental health professionals with a basic understanding that, it is hoped, will enhance their capacity to identify the cases, treat and rehabilitate them, and advocate for policies that meet their needs.

METHOD

A literature search for studies of the epidemiology of YOD used the PubMed and Google Scholar databases, searching for full-text papers written in the English language. The search terms were: "young-onset dementia" or "early-onset dementia" in combinations with "prevalence" or "incidence" or "survival" or "mortality." The references of the articles found were reviewed for additional sources and already-familiar sources were scoured, particularly topical reviews and white papers.

FREQUENCY AND DISTRIBUTION

Estimates of the frequency of YOD are scarce; data mainly derive from catchment area or specialty clinic samples, using surveys of local clinics and hospitals, medical record review, disease registries, and passive surveillance of defined geographic regions for case identification. Direct ascertainment from the population is difficult because of the rarity and diversity of YOD conditions, their diagnostic complexity (which demands expertise), and the public's lack of familiarity with these conditions (which makes surveys difficult to design).

The proportions of specialist clinic (or memory clinic) patients who suffer YOD are shown in **Table 1**. These data indicate that the frequency of YOD in specialist clinics ranges from 7.3% to 44%.[5–11] These estimates reflect differences between regions and centers in the clinical focus, local practices, referral base, and sampling methods. For example, the study conducted in Greece, which reports the highest frequency, received referrals mainly from academic psychiatrists and neurologists, which may have resulted in a case selection favoring atypical forms of dementia (and younger cases than the typical memory clinic).

The prevalence of all-cause YOD in communities is shown in **Table 2**. These studies, which typically identify cases in the catchment area of a specialist center or network, show prevalence rates ranging 42.3 to 68.2 per 100,000 at risk (ie, for adults falling into the age groups studied).[12–16] Variability results from differences between case mix (**Table 3**) and the sampling methods (one example is the differences in sample age ranges shown in **Table 2**). The incidence of all-cause YOD, based on the 3 studies conducted to date, is 11 to 13.4 per 100,000.[17–19]

ETIOLOGY

The case mix in prevalence studies of YOD is broad, comprising Alzheimer disease (AD), frontotemporal dementia (FTD), vascular dementia (VaD), Huntington disease (HD), Parkinson disease (PDD) and dementia with Lewy bodies (DLB), alcohol-related dementia (ARD), and traumatic brain injury (TBI).[5,6,8–10,12,13,15,16,20,21] AD and FTD are the most frequent neurodegenerative causes of YOD (see **Table 3** for frequencies derived from prevalence studies). In the United States, it has been estimated that 200,000 have young-onset AD[22] and between 12,000 and 18,000 have young-onset FTD.[23] Cerebrovascular disease and stroke are important causes of YOD in Japan.[13] Neurodegenerative causes of YOD predominate beyond age 35,[21] and it has been estimated that they comprise 30% of all YOD.[24] TBI, ARD, and human immunodeficiency virus–associated neurocognitive disorder are mainly seen among the poor living in inner cities.[6]

Table 1
Frequency of YOD dementia in specialized clinics

Study/Year	Location	Study Population	Case Ascertainment	YOD/Total	% YOD
Yokota et al,[5] 2005	Okayama, Japan	Outpatient clinic	Referrals from generalists, neurologists, and psychiatrists	34/464	7.3
McMurtray et al,[6] 2006	Los Angeles, CA	Memory center	Medical records	278/1683	30
Shinagawa et al,[7] 2007	Ehime, Japan	Memory clinic	Referrals from generalists, geriatricians, and neuropsychiatrists	185/861	27.7
Nandi et al,[8] 2008	West Bengal, India	Specialized clinic	Medical records	94/379	24.5
Papageorgiou et al,[9] 2009	Athens, Greece	Specialized center	Referrals from neurologists and psychiatrists	114/260	44
Picard et al,[10] 2011	Amiens, Lille, and Rouen, France	Cohort of 3 memory clinics	Referrals	811/3473	23.5
Croisile et al,[11] 2012	Lyons, France	Memory clinic	Referrals	91/746	12.2

Table 2
Frequency of YOD (all causes) in geographic populations

Prevalence Studies

Study/Year	Location	Study Population	Case Ascertainment	Age, Years	Prevalence[a]	95% CI
Harvey et al,[12] 2003	London, UK	Catchment area	Registry and surveillance of local practices	35–64	54	45.1–64.1
Ikejima et al,[13] 2009	Ibaraki, Japan	Regional network	Postal survey to clinics, hospitals, nursing facilities, and health agencies	20–64	42.3	39.4–45.4
Borroni et al,[14] 2011	Brescia County, Italy	Regional network of hospital-based centers	Disease registry	45–65	55.1	47.0–63.4
Renvoize et al,[15] 2011	Blackpool, Wyre, and Fylde, UK	Catchment area	Medical records	45–64	62.8	48.0–82.3
Withall et al,[16] 2014	Eastern Sydney, Australia	Catchment area	Structured questionnaire to health professionals, and medical records	30–64	68.2	54.9–83.4

Incidence Studies

Study/Year	Location	Study Population	Case Ascertainment	Age (y)	Incidence[a]	95% CI
Mercy et al,[17] 2008	Cambridgeshire, UK	Catchment area	Referrals from generalists and specialists	45–64	11.5	8.6–15.0
Garre-Olmo et al,[18] 2010	Catalonia, Spain	Regional network of hospitals	Standardized clinical registry	30–64	13.4	11.3–15.8
Sanchez Abraham et al,[19] 2014	Mar del Plata, Argentina	Hospital serving large catchment area	Database of geriatric care department	<65	11	6.25–19.1

[a] per 100,000 persons at risk.

Table 3
Frequency of YOD by etiologic type

	Location	N	Age Range[a]	Age, Onset[a]	Age, Exam[a]	AD	FTD	VaD	HD	DLB/PDD	ARD	TBI
Ferran et al,[20] 1996	Liverpool, North Wales, Cheshire, and Lancashire, UK	200	<65	52.6	56	27	4	17	NR	2	12	NR
Harvey et al,[12] 2003	London, UK	185	30–65	NR	58.7	34	12	18	4.9	7.5	10	EX
Yokota et al,[5] 2005	Okayama, Japan	34	<65	NR	NR	38.8	14.7	23.5	NR	2.9	NR	NR
McMurtray et al,[6] 2006	Los Angeles, CA	278	<65	51.5	56.5	17	3	29	NR	NR	5	24
Kelley et al,[21] 2008	Rochester, USA	235	17–45	34.7	36.7	1.7	13.2	5.9	7.7	0.4	0.4	EX
Nandi et al,[8] 2008	West Bengal, India	94	<65	56.5	NR	33	27	20	4	4	NR	NR
Ikejima et al,[13] 2009	Ibaraki, Japan	617	20–64	53.4	NR	25.6	2.8	42.5	NR	6.2	NR	7.1
Papageorgiou et al,[9] 2009	Athens, Greece	114	<65	55.1	58.7	27.2	24.6	6.1	2.6	4.4	NR	0.87
Picard et al,[10] 2011	Amiens, Lille, and Rouen, France	811	<65	55.9	NR	22.3	79.7	15.9	3	5.3	9.4	3.8
Renvoize et al,[15] 2011	Blackpool, Wyre, and Fylde, UK	55	<65	NR	NR	24.2	2.4	6.0	2.4	1.2	10.9	NR
Withall et al,[16] 2014	Eastern Sydney, Australia	141	<65	55	56.5	17.7	11.3	12.8	5.7	4.9	18.4	2.1

Some causes are not shown here (owing to focus, limited coverage in the reports, small numbers, and space limits): dementia associated with depression (18% of cases in Ferran et al,[20] 1996), corticobasal degeneration, progressive supranuclear palsy, Creutzfeldt-Jakob disease, depression, cerebral tumor, multiple sclerosis, human immunodeficiency virus infection, epilepsy, and unspecified types.

Abbreviations: EX, the condition was an exclusion criterion; NR, data pertaining to the variable were not reported.

[a] Age variables are in years; means are reported for age of onset and age at examination (or at ascertainment). Age range refers to the reference range for the study. Frequencies are reported as percentages of the sample for ease of comparison.

RISK FACTORS

Hereditary transmission is the most established risk factor for neurodegenerative forms of YOD. Hereditary forms of AD and FTD arise from autosomal dominant mutations in several genetic loci (**Table 4**, which also shows data for Huntington disease and prion disease). Mutations in specific genetic loci are often associated with phenotypic variants, as described in **Table 4**. For example, the mutation in the C9ORF72 gene gives rise to a phenotype of FTD with amyotrophic lateral sclerosis (FTD-ALS), which is often also heralded or complicated by psychosis.

Repeated concussive head traumas, typically sustained in sports such as boxing, American football, and ice hockey, are now known to cause chronic traumatic encephalopathy, a neurodegenerative dementia[25] characterized by widespread cortical and subcortical tauopathy. Low cognition, alcohol abuse, high blood pressure, stroke, depression, and neuroleptic use in youth were linked to YOD in one study.[26] Another study found association between YOD and cardiovascular disease (eg, stroke, transient ischemic attack, chronic kidney disease, and hypertension).[27] These findings suggest opportunities for primary prevention.[28]

SURVIVAL

Life expectancy after diagnosis varies widely in YOD, according to the etiologic type, but appears to be shorter in general than for late-onset dementia.[29] It is estimated that median survival from diagnosis for YOD (derived from a study that focused on AD and VaD cases) is 6 years.[30] Median survival from diagnosis of FTD is about 7 to 13 years in clinic cohorts and 6 to 8 years in neuropathologic series.[31] Survival is much shorter in FTD-ALS, showing median survival of 27 months.[32] Survival in prion disease cases is comparable to that in FTD-ALS, although some cases survive up to 2 to 3 years.[33]

CLINICAL AND DIAGNOSTIC CONSIDERATIONS

The diagnosis of YOD is frequently missed because of the wide diversity of types, a predominance of nonmemory and neuropsychiatric features in many, and (relative to late-onset dementia) a high frequency of syndromes that are defined by motor dysfunctions such as Parkinsonism, apraxia, and ataxia.

When certain diagnostic principles are followed, which derive from a clinical epidemiology that defines syndromes according to their signal phenomena, the differential diagnosis can be sharply narrowed. Diagnosis entails an algorithmic approach, not as a sequence of procedures but in the sense of a methodical consideration of the clinical data. The key data elements are the cluster of cognitive, neuropsychiatric, and motor symptoms and signs defining a syndrome, their chronology and tempo, and family history (particularly of neuropsychiatric and neurologic illnesses). These data guide what diagnostic procedures are selected—psychometric measurements, serologic and biochemical assays, brain imaging, and genotyping—and facilitates their interpretation. This approach is illustrated in **Fig. 1**, which presents an algorithmic approach for using syndrome type (defined from the most salient symptoms and signs) to progressively narrow the differential diagnosis.

DIFFERENTIAL DIAGNOSIS AS A FUNCTION OF DEFINED SYNDROMES

The first branch point in our algorithm (see **Fig. 1**) involves weighing the chronology and tempo of the illness. An insidious, ingravescent course is typical of most neurodegenerative disorders, including AD, FTD, HD, and DLB, and is also true of some presentations of VaD.[34] An abrupt and rapid development can arise from some

Table 4
Genetic loci for common neurodegenerative disorders

	Gene	Locus	Clinical Feature
Alzheimer's disease	PSEN1	14q24	Often resembles sporadic AD; however, behavior presentation (agitation, depression, delusions, and hallucinations) and motor symptoms (myoclonus, spastic paresis, Parkinsonism, seizures) are prominent in some cases.
	PSEN 2	1q31	Rare (typically Volga German ancestry). Most commonly presents with amnesia. There is a high degree of phenotypic variation, 33% presenting with hallucinations and delusions and 31% with seizures. Disease progression is slow, with rigidity, mutism, and a bedridden state in the end stages.
	APP	21q21	Amnesic dementia associated with seizures commonly developing within 1 to 9 y after onset of dementia. Intracerebral hemorrhage is not uncommon.
Frontotemporal dementia	C9ORF72	9p21	Behavioral dementia (FTD) with ALS
	MAPT	17q21	Behavioral dementia with Parkinsonism
	GRN	17q21	Behavioral dementia, with aphasia, apraxia, Parkinsonism, and dystonia
	VCP	9p13	Inclusion body myopathy with osteolytic bone disease (Paget's disease) and behavioral dementia
	CHMP2B	3p11.2	Very rare, seen in Danish kindred; behavioral dementia, Parkinsonism, and progressive spastic paresis are often seen.
Huntington disease	Huntington	4p16	Choreoathetosis early in the course, with dystonia and akinetic rigidity in later stages. Neuropsychiatric features include executive dysfunction, depression, irritability, impulsivity, compulsive behaviors, anger and hostility, and depression.
Prion disease	PRNP	20p13	Accounts for 15% of human prion disease. Several types are recognized: fCJD, which in rare instances mimics amnesic AD, typically features myoclonic jerks, cerebellar signs, and akinetic mutism; FFI (progressive insomnia, dysautonomia, selective thalamic degeneration); GSS (a hereditary form with chronic cerebellar ataxia), pyramidal features, dysarthria, ocular dysmetria, and hyporeflexia, with dementia in later stages.

Abbreviations: APP, amyloid precursor protein; C9ORF72, chromosome 9 open reading frame 72; CHMP2B, chromatin-modifying protein 2B; f CJD, familial CJD; FFI, familial fatal insomnia; GRN, progranulin; GSS, Gerstmann-Straussler-Sheinker syndrome; MAPT, microtubule-associated protein tau; PRNP, prion protein; PSEN, presenilin; VCP, valosin-containing protein.

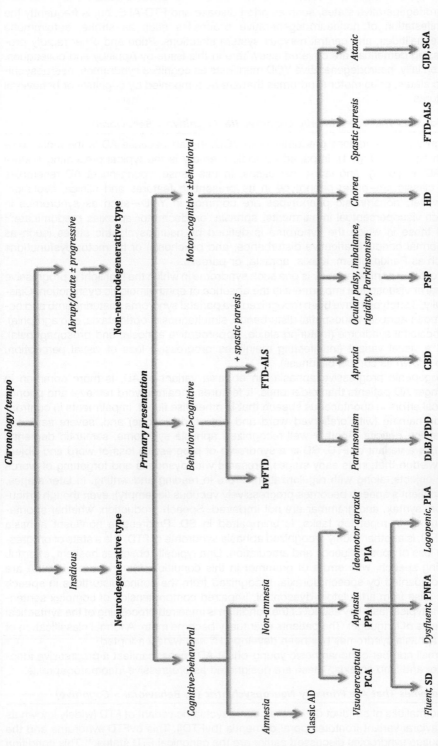

Fig. 1. Algorithm for discriminating the neurodegenerative types of YOD. PCA, posterior cortical atrophy; PIA, progressive ideomotor apraxia; PLA, progressive logopenic aphasia; PPA, primary progressive aphasia; PNFA, progressive non-fluent aphasia; PSP, progressive supranuclear palsy; SCA, spinocerebellar ataxia.

neurodegenerative states, such as prion disease and FTD-ALS, but is frequently the manifestation of nonneurodegenerative processes such as stroke, autoimmune encephalitides, and central nervous system infections. Prion and other rapidly progressing dementias are covered elsewhere in this issue by Appleby and colleagues. Essentially, neurodegenerative YOD manifests as cognitive syndromes, neuropsychiatric states, or as motor syndromes that are accompanied by cognitive or behavioral features.

Syndromes That Are Primarily Cognitive (ie, Cognitive > Behavioral)

Cognitive presentations predominate in YOD, in part because AD is the most common type (see **Fig. 1**). Impaired episodic memory is the typical presenting feature of AD, in young- and late-onset cases. In this sense, young-onset AD resembles the classic late-onset phenotype in its presenting features and clinical evolution. However, nonamnesic phenotypes are common in YOD—such as syndromes in which visuoperceptual impairments, aphasia, or ideomotor apraxias predominate[35] and those in which the syndrome is defined by neuropsychiatric states (such as abnormal conduct, affective disturbance, and psychosis) or by motor dysfunctions (such as Parkinsonism, ataxia, apraxia, or paresis).

Posterior cortical atrophy is one such syndrome in which the highlight is progressive visual or visuospatial impairment in the absence of ophthalmologic dysfunction. Classically, 3 subtypes have been recognized—a parietal syndrome (featuring limb and oculomotor apraxia, visuospatial disturbance, simultagnosia, optic ataxia, and agraphia), an occipital syndrome (featuring alexia, apperceptive agnosia, and prosopagnosia), and a visual variant (manifesting mainly as progressive loss of visual perception, also known as cortical blindness).

Logopenic progressive aphasia, an aphasia variant of AD, is more common in younger AD patients than older ones. It features impaired word retrieval and phonological errors in spontaneous speech that is otherwise fluent, impairments in confrontation naming (with preserved word and object knowledge) and, severe sentence repetition deficits. Another well-recognized aphasia syndrome, semantic dementia (SD), is a variant of FTD. SD is a syndrome of progressive loss of word and object knowledge that, in its early stages, presents with dysnomia and forgetting of words and objects, along with regularization errors in reading and writing. In later stages, the patient's speech becomes progressively vacuous (ie, empty), even though articulation, syntax, and grammar are not impaired. Speech production, whether spontaneous or in repetition tasks, is unimpaired in SD. Progressive nonfluent aphasia (PNFA), is another widely recognized aphasia syndrome of FTD. It is a state of progressive loss of speech fluency and articulation. One typically observes hesitant, effortful, halting speech, with errors of grammar in this condition. Many cases of PNFA are accompanied by speech apraxia, recognized from the sound distortions in speech that arise from articulatory dyscontrol. Impaired comprehension of complex sentences is typical (as a key aspect of the condition is impaired processing of the syntactical aspects of language). The patients eventually become mute. A formal classification of the aphasia syndromes has been developed[36] and widely adopted.

Small number of nonamnesic young-onset AD cases manifest a progressive ideomotor and limb apraxia. These are designated as progressive ideomotor apraxia.

Syndromes That Are Primarily Neuropsychiatric (ie, Behavioral > Cognitive)

Abnormalities of conduct define the neuropsychiatric variant of FTD (widely known as behavioral variant frontotemporal dementia [bvFTD]). This bvFTD syndrome and the language syndromes discussed earlier are the canonical FTD states.[37] This condition manifests as a progressive coarsening of temperament, judgment, conduct, and social skills and derangements of volition. Formal diagnostic criteria have been developed.[38] It is not uncommon for bvFTD to be accompanied by a progressive spastic paresis, in which case the condition is known as FTD-ALS. Parkinsonism can also accompany it, but the condition is primarily a derangement of behavior.

Syndromes Defined by Motor Dysfunction (ie, Motor Disorder > Cognitive/Behavioral)

These syndromes are defined by motor dysfunction, such as Parkinsonism, motor apraxia, dyscontrol, spastic paresis, abnormalities of posture and gait, chorea, or ataxia. DLB and PDD overlap in their clinical and pathologic features, differing primarily in the order of emergence of Parkinsonism and dementia, and in the symmetry of the former (lateral asymmetry is typical of Parkinson disease). In DLB, dementia precedes Parkinsonism, or both states emerge simultaneously (or in close temporal proximity). Generally in PDD, dementia does not appear in the first decade of the illness, although formal neuropsychological assessment may uncover subclinical executive dysfunction in some patients in the early stages. Dementia is a central feature of DLB. Parkinsonism is also a core feature of the syndrome. Dementia arising within 1 year after Parkinsonism is the convention for separating DLB from PDD.[39] Rest tremor is uncommon common in DLB, whereas it is seen in most PDD cases. As noted earlier, lateral asymmetry is typical of PDD. Axial tendency, more pronounced masked facies, postural instability, and gait disorder in DLB are additional features that facilitate distinguishing the 2 conditions.[39] DLB and PDD show fluctuations of alertness, attention and mentation, and recurrent formed visual hallucinations. Paranoia and delusions are not uncommon either.

Chorea and dyskinesias are typical of adult-onset HD. Chorea is the most prominent feature and appears early. Ataxia, bradykinesia, and rigidity are mainly seen in juvenile and young-adult presentations of HD. Executive dysfunction, behavioral rigidity, irritability, and flighty emotions are also early features[40,41] but are overshadowed by the dramatic motor phenomena.

Corticobasal degeneration (CBD) and progressive supranuclear palsy (PSP) have overlapping clinical and pathologic features. CBD features asymmetric limb apraxia, akinesia, rigidity, dystonia, oral buccal apraxia, dysarticulation of speech (speech apraxia), and dysarthria. Executive dysfunction, which develops early, is overshadowed by these motor phenomena. Many patients have the behavioral and language dysfunctions associated with FTD during the illness.[42] PSP features oculomotor palsy, postural instability with retropulsion (ie, a tendency to fall backwards), executive dysfunction, behavioral dyscontrol, apathy, depression, and symmetric Parkinsonian features (rigidity, tremor, hypo/bradykinesia).

Amyotrophic lateral sclerosis (ALS) commonly features cognitive impairments, being accompanied by executive dysfunction and aphasia, and by FTD syndromes in a subset.[43] This phenomenon is now known to be linked to mutation of the C9ORF72 gene.[44,45] ALS features progressive limb or pharyngeal spasticity, muscle wasting and fasciculations, and paresis (progressing to paralysis). Many cases manifest emotional dysfunction, characterized by involuntary or hair-trigger laughing and crying (the so-called pseudobulbar effect).

Most cases of Creutzfeldt-Jakob disease (CJD) are sporadic forms (ie, sCJD). sCJD is a rapidly progressive dementia manifesting some combination of ataxia, myoclonus, cortical blindness, motor dyscontrol, spasticity, incoordination, Parkinsonism, and akinetic mutism. Several atypical forms are recognized: an ataxic CJD in which loss of coordination predominates, a visuoperceptual variant that culminates in cortical blindness, an amyotrophic variant featuring progressive spastic paresis and progressive muscle atrophy, and an encephalopathic type featuring rapidly progressive dementia with myoclonus and akinetic mutism. CJD may also present with a predominance of cognitive impairments (mainly amnesia, disorientation and apraxia) or as a primary neuropsychiatric state featuring depression, anxiety, and agitation.[46]

Spinocerebellar ataxias are a family of hereditary cerebellar degenerations manifesting progressive ataxia and incoordination, accompanied by dysarthria and dysphagia. They can be distinguished from ataxic CJD states by their gradual evolution, typically spanning a few decades. Executive dysfunction, cognitive dysmetria, and affective lability can be seen in many cases.[47] Dementia is not universal, but severe dysarthria, motor incoordination, incontinence, and dyscontrol of cognition and affect can mimic a mild dementia.

VaD is not depicted in **Fig. 1**; it is not neurodegenerative. When it arises from overt stroke, the diagnosis is straightforward. Generally the clinical picture is variable, as it depends on the mechanism and distribution of the cerebrovascular disease underlying its development. Although VaD is common after stroke, it may follow relatively

---

Box 1
Characteristics, symptoms, and signs that suggest neurodegenerative etiology of a psychiatric state

- Historical
  - Later than typical age at onset
  - Puzzling atypical features
  - Family history of dementia, Parkinsonism, or other motor disorder
  - Unusual prodrome, eg, insomnia, hyperphagia
  - Rapid evolution
- Mental status
  - Poor insight
  - Apathy/indifference
  - Compulsions without obsessions
  - Visual hallucinations
- Cognitive symptoms
  - Aphasia
  - Apraxia
  - Visual complaints (other than hallucinations)
  - Spatial disorientation
  - Incontinence
- Physical/motor signs
  - Abnormal posture and movement
  - Frequent falls at early stage
  - Frequent (myoclonic) jerking
  - Progressive motor weakness
  - Declining motor coordination
  - Left-right asymmetry

small infarcts in strategic locations or arise from chronic cerebrovascular insufficiency.[34] Thus, VaD may arise as a sudden and catastrophic crippling of cognitive, mental, and motor functions after hemorrhagic stroke; as the classical stepwise decline in cognition accompanied by behavioral and motor phenomena; or as a hemiplegic or hemiparetic state with focal cognitive deficits (typically a nonfluent aphasia). Some cases show an insidious progression that is difficult to distinguish from AD, FTD, or DLB. The classical presentation is characterized by executive dysfunction, affective dyscontrol (typically emotional incontinence), psychomotor slowing, motor dyscontrol, Parkinsonism, imbalance, and a gait impairment (small-step, apraxic, or Parkinsonian gait).[34,48]

MEASUREMENT AND SCREENING FOR CASE DETECTION

Measurement is fundamental to neuropsychiatry practice, serving different goals, such as case detection (ie, screening), differential diagnosis, and monitoring. Currently, there are no practical methods for screening for cases in the community. Proposals for screening for dementia in primary care have typically focused on late-life cases of amnesic dementia (ie, late-onset AD), and are not likely to be practical for screening for YOD, owing to the diversity of presentations, overlap with primary psychiatric disorders (including major depression, bipolar disorder, and obsessive compulsive disorder) and the variety of settings in which the cases present, such as primary care, psychiatry settings, and neurology clinics. Furthermore, bedside instruments such as the Mini Mental State Examination (MMSE) are not suitable for this population because many cases, particularly those in which neuropsychiatric phenomena define the phenotype, can attain scores matching those attained by their counterparts who either have normal cognitive function or subclinical impairments.[49]

A practical approach to screening psychiatric populations for cases of neurodegenerative disease involves identifying red flags,[50] features that serve as indicators that the syndrome of interest may be a neurodegenerative mimic rather than a primary psychiatric state. These red flags are depicted in **Box 1**. Formal measurement methods, and their application to differential diagnosis and monitoring of progression, are covered elsewhere in this issue by Harciarek and colleagues.

SUMMARY

YODs are topical for psychiatry because of the syndromes, their psychological and psychosocial aspects, and the skillset of the psychiatrist. Psychiatrists have a role to play in the diagnosis of these conditions and in their management. Understanding the clinical epidemiology aids in the diagnosis of these conditions. Appreciating the varied etiologic distribution—the cognitive, neuropsychiatric, and motor syndromes, and the clinical genetic epidemiology—allows the physician with a high index of suspicion to apply a methodical approach to identifying potential cases, distinguishing them from primary psychiatric conditions, and making a specific diagnosis.

REFERENCES

1. van Vliet D, de Vugt ME, Bakker C, et al. Time to diagnosis in young-onset dementia as compared with late-onset dementia. Psychol Med 2013;43: 423–32.
2. van Vliet D, de Vugt ME, Bakker C, et al. Impact of early onset dementia on caregivers: a review. Int J Geriatr Psychiatry 2010;25:1091–100.

3. Rosenthal Gelman C, Greer C. Young children in early-onset alzheimer's disease families: research gaps and emerging service needs. Am J Alzheimers Dis Other Demen 2011;26:29–35.

4. Millenaar JK, van Vliet D, Bakker C, et al. The experiences and needs of children living with a parent with young onset dementia: results from the NeedYD study. Int Psychogeriatr 2014;26:2001–10.

5. Yokota O, Sasaki K, Fujisawa Y, et al. Frequency of early and late-onset dementias in a Japanese memory disorders clinic. Eur J Neurol 2005;12:782–90.

6. McMurtray A, Clark D, Christine D, et al. Early-onset dementia: frequency and causes compared to late-onset dementia. Dement Geriatr Cogn Disord 2006; 21:59–64.

7. Shinagawa S, Ikeda M, Toyota Y, et al. Frequency and clinical characteristics of early-onset dementia in consecutive patients in a memory clinic. Dement Geriatr Cogn Disord 2007;24:42–7.

8. Nandi SP, Biswas A, Pal S, et al. Clinical profile of young-onset dementia: A study from Eastern India. Neurol Asia 2008;13:103–8.

9. Papageorgiou SG, Kontaxis T, Bonakis A, et al. Frequency and causes of early-onset dementia in a tertiary referral center in Athens. Alzheimer Dis Assoc Disord 2009;23:347–51.

10. Picard C, Pasquier F, Martinaud O, et al. Early onset dementia: characteristics in a large cohort from academic memory clinics. Alzheimer Dis Assoc Disord 2011; 25:203–5.

11. Croisile B, Tedesco A, Bernard E, et al. Diagnostic profile of young-onset dementia before 65 years. Experience of a french memory referral center. Rev Neurol (Paris) 2012;168:161–9 [in French].

12. Harvey R, Skelton-Robinson M, Rossor M. The prevalence and causes of dementia in people under the age of 65 years. J Neurol Neurosurg Psychiatry 2003;74: 1206–9.

13. Ikejima C, Yasuno F, Mizukami K, et al. Prevalence and causes of early-onset dementia in Japan: a population-based study. Stroke 2009;40:2709–14.

14. Borroni B, Alberici A, Grassi M, et al. Prevalence and demographic features of early-onset neurodegenerative dementia in Brescia county, Italy. Alzheimer Dis Assoc Disord 2011;25:341–4.

15. Renvoize E, Hanson M, Dale M. Prevalence and causes of young onset dementia in an English health district. Int J Geriatr Psychiatry 2011;26:106–7.

16. Withall A, Draper B, Seeher K, et al. The prevalence and causes of younger onset dementia in Eastern Sydney, Australia. Int Psychogeriatr 2014;26:1955–65.

17. Mercy L, Hodges JR, Dawson K, et al. Incidence of early-onset dementias in Cambridgeshire, United Kingdom. Neurology 2008;71:1496–9.

18. Garre-Olmo J, Genís Batlle D, del Mar Fernández M, et al. Incidence and subtypes of early-onset dementia in a geographically defined general population. Neurology 2010;75:1249–55.

19. Sanchez Abraham M, Scharovsky D, Romano LM, et al. Incidence of early-onset dementia in Mar del Plata. Neurologia 2014. http://dx.doi.org/10.1016/j.nrl.2013. 10.009.

20. Ferran J, Wilson K, Doran M, et al. The early onset dementias: a study of clinical characteristics and service use. Int J Geriatr Psychiatry 1996;11:863–9.

21. Kelley B, Boeve BF, Josephs K. Young-onset dementia: demographic and etiologic characteristics of 235 patients. Arch Neurol 2008;65:1502–8.

22. Alzheimer's Association. 2014 Alzheimer's disease facts and figures. Alzheimers Demen 2014;10:e47–92.

23. Knopman DS, Roberts RO. Estimating the number of persons with frontotemporal lobar degeneration in the US population. J Mol Neurosci 2011;45:330–5.
24. Kuruppu DK, Matthews BR. Young-onset dementia. Semin Neurol 2013;33:365–85.
25. Baugh CM, Stamm JM, Riley DO, et al. Chronic traumatic encephalopathy: neuro-degeneration following repetitive concussive and subconcussive brain trauma. Brain Imaging Behav 2012;6:244–54.
26. Nordström P, Nordström A, Eriksson M, et al. Risk factors in late adolescence for young-onset dementia in men: a nationwide cohort study. JAMA Intern Med 2013; 173:1612–8.
27. Heath CA, Mercer SW, Guthrie B. Vascular comorbidities in younger people with dementia: a cross-sectional population-based study of 616 245 middle-aged people in Scotland. J Neurol Neurosurg Psychiatry 2014. http://dx.doi.org/10. 1136/jnnp-2014-309033.
28. Onyike CU. In young men, various risk factors are associated with later development of young-onset dementia. Evid Based Ment Health 2014;17:49.
29. Koedam EL, Pijnenburg YA, Deeg DJ, et al. Early-onset dementia is associated with higher mortality. Dement Geriatr Cogn Disord 2008;26:147–52.
30. Kay DW, Forster DP, Newens AJ. Long-term survival, place of death, and death certification in clinically diagnosed pre-senile dementia in northern England Follow-up after 8-12 years. Br J Psychiatry 2000;177:156–62.
31. Onyike CU. What is the life expectancy in frontotemporal lobar degeneration? Neuroepidemiology 2011;37:166–7.
32. Hu WT, Seelaar H, Josephs KA, et al. Survival profiles of patients with frontotemporal dementia and motor neuron disease. Arch Neurol 2009;66:1359–64.
33. Appleby BS, Lyketsos CG. Rapidly progressive dementias and the treatment of human prion diseases. Expert Opin Pharmacother 2011;12:1–12.
34. Onyike CU. Cerebrovascular disease and dementia. Int Rev Psychiatry 2006;18: 423–31.
35. Mendez MF. Early-onset Alzheimer's disease: nonamnestic subtypes and type 2 AD. Arch Med Res 2012;43:677–85.
36. Gorno-Tempini ML, Hillis AE, Weintraub S, et al. Classification of primary progressive aphasia and its variants. Neurology 2011;76:1006–14.
37. Neary D, Snowden JS, Gustafson L, et al. Frontotemporal lobar degeneration: a consensus on clinical diagnostic criteria. Neurology 1998;51:1546–54.
38. Rascovsky K, Hodges JR, Knopman D, et al. Sensitivity of revised diagnostic criteria for the behavioural variant of frontotemporal dementia. Brain 2011;134: 2456–77.
39. McKeith IG, Dickson DW, Lowe J, et al. Diagnosis and management of dementia with Lewy bodies: third report of the DLB Consortium. Neurology 2005;65:1863–72.
40. Rosenblatt A, Leroi I. Neuropsychiatry of Huntington's disease and other basal ganglia disorders. Psychosomatics 2000;41:24–30.
41. Rosenblatt A. Understanding the psychiatric prodrome of Huntington disease. J Neurol Neurosurg Psychiatry 2007;78:913.
42. Kertesz A, Blair M, McMonagle P, et al. The diagnosis and course of frontotemporal dementia. Alzheimer Dis Assoc Disord 2007;21:155–63.
43. Bak T, Hodges JR. Cognition, language and behaviour in motor neurone disease: evidence of frontotemporal dysfunction. Dement Geriatr Cogn Disord 1999; 10(Suppl 1):29–32.
44. DeJesus-Hernandez M, Mackenzie IR, Boeve BF, et al. Expanded GGGGCC Hexanucleotide Repeat in Noncoding Region of C9ORF72 Causes Chromosome 9p-Linked FTD and ALS. Neuron 2011;72:245–56.

45. Renton AE, Majounie E, Waite A, et al. A Hexanucleotide Repeat Expansion in C9ORF72 Is the Cause of Chromosome 9p21-Linked ALS-FTD. Neuron 2011; 72:257–68.
46. Appleby BS, Appleby KK, Crain BJ, et al. Characteristics of established and proposed sporadic Creutzfeldt-Jakob disease variants. Arch Neurol 2009;66: 208–15.
47. Schmahmann JD. Disorders of the cerebellum: ataxia, dysmetria of thought, and the cerebellar cognitive affective syndrome. J Neuropsychiatry Clin Neurosci 2004;16:367–78.
48. Ridha B, Josephs K. Young-onset dementia: a practical approach to diagnosis. Neurologist 2006;12:2–13.
49. Onyike CU, Sloane KL, Smyth SF, et al. Estimating severity of illness and disability in frontotemporal dementia: preliminary analysis of the Dementia Disability Rating (DDR). Acta Neuropsychol 2011;9:141–53.
50. Wylie MA, Shnall A, Onyike CU, et al. Management of frontotemporal dementia in mental health and multidisciplinary settings. Int Rev Psychiatry 2013;25:230–6.

The Neuropsychiatric Examination of the Young-Onset Dementias

Simon Ducharme, MD, MSc[a,b,*], Bradford C. Dickerson, MD[c,d]

KEYWORDS

- Neuropsychiatry • Young-onset dementia • Early onset dementia
- Frontotemporal dementia • Alzheimer disease • Differential diagnosis • Biomarkers

KEY POINTS

- Young-onset dementias often present with prominent behavioral features; the differential diagnosis includes a large number of medical, neurologic, and psychiatric disorders. Psychiatrists play a key role in identifying patients suffering from one of these conditions.
- Frontotemporal dementia (FTD) constitutes a significant proportion of cases of young-onset dementias. This condition includes the behavioral variant of FTD featuring clinical symptoms that have a striking overlap with many primary psychiatric disorders.
- The neuropsychiatric assessment of young-onset dementias starts with a detailed history of the nature and longitudinal progression of symptoms. A knowledgeable informant should be interviewed in all cases.
- The clinical assessment and biomarkers, including neuroimaging, cerebrospinal fluid, and genetics, can be integrated in a probabilistic model to determine the most likely neuropathology underlying a clinical syndrome.

INTRODUCTION

Young-onset dementias (<65 years old) constitute 20% to 30% of all dementia cases seen in specialty clinics[1–3] but a much smaller proportion of all dementias because most elderly patients are not followed in those clinics. Incidence has been estimated

Disclosure: Dr S. Ducharme has no disclosure or conflict of interest to report. Dr B.C. Dickerson is a consultant for Merck, Inc, Forum Pharmaceuticals, Inc, and the Med Learning Group, Inc.
[a] Department of Psychiatry, McGill University Health Centre and Montreal Neurological Institute, McGill University, 3801 University Street, Montreal, Quebec H3A 2B4, Canada; [b] McConnell Brain Imaging Centre, Montreal Neurological Institute, McGill University, 3801 University Street, Montreal, Quebec H3A 2B4, Canada; [c] MGH FTD Unit, Massachusetts General Hospital, 149 13th Street, Suite 2691, Charlestown, MA 02129, USA; [d] Department of Neurology, Harvard Medical School, 25 Shattuck Street, Boston, MA 02115, USA
* Corresponding author. Department of Psychiatry, McGill University Health Centre and Montreal Neurological Institute, McGill University, 3801 University Street, Montreal, Quebec H3A 2B4, Canada.
E-mail address: simon.ducharme@mcgill.ca

Psychiatr Clin N Am 38 (2015) 249–264
http://dx.doi.org/10.1016/j.psc.2015.01.002
psych.theclinics.com

Abbreviations	
ACE	Addenbrooke's Cognitive Examination
AD	Alzheimer disease
ADL	Activities of daily living
ALS	Amyotrophic lateral sclerosis
bvFTD	Behavioral variant frontotemporal dementia
CSF	Cerebrospinal fluid
EEG	Electroencephalography
FTD	Frontotemporal dementia
FTLD	Frontotemporal lobar degeneration
MoCA	Montreal Cognitive Assessment
NMDA	N-methyl-d-aspartate
PCA	Posterior cortical atrophy
PD	Parkinson disease
PPA	Primary progressive aphasia

at 13.4 cases per 100,000 person-years,[4] with a higher incidence (up to 113 out of 100,000) in the age range closer to 65 years.[5] Young-onset dementias are common enough to be encountered in a variety of clinical settings and present a diagnostic challenge for clinicians for a few reasons.[6] By definition these neurodegenerative diseases occur at an age in which the degree of a priori suspicion for dementia is low, which can lead to missed cases. In younger patients clinical manifestations tend to be disproportionately more behavioral than cognitive, which can also steer clinicians away from the correct diagnosis.[6] Because of the combination of these two factors, patients are often first seen in primary care medicine or general psychiatric settings in which young-onset dementia is rare. Although these clinicians can play a key role in identifying and evaluating early signs and symptoms of young-onset dementia, they typically have little experience working with this population. This article reviews the steps and structure of the neuropsychiatric assessment for young-onset dementia, focusing on key elements of the history-taking process, examination, office-based cognitive testing, and differential diagnosis. The use of neuropsychological testing, neuroimaging, and genetics is discussed; but these topics are covered in more detail by Harciarek and colleagues, Goldman, and Shim and colleagues in other articles in this issue.

GENERAL PRINCIPLES

In order to perform the neuropsychiatric assessment of young-onset dementias, clinicians need to have a broad knowledge of the symptoms that can be observed in the various subtypes of dementia and how those can be differentiated from other general medical, neurologic, and psychiatric disorders. Indeed, young-onset dementias can produce a wide variety of behavioral, cognitive, and neurologic symptoms. Although the prototypical form of each neurocognitive clinical syndrome has specific core features, many patients do not follow all the rules and some of these features, especially when considered individually, may overlap substantially with other neurologic and psychiatric disorders. This overlap happens because symptoms are related to the anatomic pattern of cerebral atrophy/dysfunction and its impact on distributed neuronal networks. In other words, symptoms are related to the anatomic distribution of the pathologic process rather than the specific pathologic process itself. As an example, a frontal distribution of Alzheimer disease (AD) pathology (ie, amyloid plaques and neurofibrillary tangles containing hyperphosphorylated tau protein) will produce behavioral symptoms similar to the clinical syndrome of behavioral variant frontotemporal dementia (bvFTD),[7] which is usually associated with tau or 43kDa TAR DNA-binding protein (TDP-43) protein aggregates.[8] A frontal brain tumor may present with similar symptoms. Moreover, symptoms of young-onset dementia can overlap with primary psychiatric disorders, especially if they involve similar neural circuitry (eg, disruption of the orbitofrontal cortex in bvFTD and obsessive-compulsive disorder).

Given that different pathologic subtypes of young-onset dementia can have overlapping clinical phenotypes (and the nonfeasibility of brain biopsy in most cases), clinicians must rely on probabilistic diagnostic models. Once the presence of a major neurocognitive disorder (dementia) is established, clinicians can estimate the level of probability of various subtypes of dementia using clinical criteria and biomarkers. The degree of certainty depends on the specificity of the clinical syndrome (eg, high probability of Lewy body dementia in a patient with a combination of visual hallucinations, cognitive fluctuations, and parkinsonism) and the results of investigations (eg, a specific genetic mutation can confirm the nature of a pathologic process). As an example, the contemporary research criteria (Rascovsky and colleagues,[9] 2011) for bvFTD have established a hierarchy of diagnostic confidence (ie, *possible*, *probable*, or *definite* bvFTD) incorporating neuroimaging features as well as genetics into the diagnostic process. A similar process was applied in the latest revision of the diagnostic criteria for AD.[10]

CAUSES AND DIFFERENTIAL DIAGNOSIS

The distribution of dementia subtypes is different in the young-onset population compared with older-age dementia.[2] Although AD probably remains the most common cause, it constitutes a smaller proportion of cases compared with late-onset cases.[1–4] In patients younger than 65 years, FTD, including bvFTD and the language variants of FTD (primary progressive aphasias [PPA]), constitutes a much higher proportion of cases and is potentially the second most common cause of dementia.[11] Vascular dementia is another common cause.[1,3] Lewy body dementia is much less common before 65 years of age compared with the geriatric population. Other nonneurodegenerative causes are also more common in frequency in the early onset population, including dementia secondary to traumatic brain injury, alcohol-related toxicity, or encephalitis.[2,3]

Among the causes of young-onset dementia, bvFTD is particularly relevant for general psychiatrists. A *Diagnostic and Statistical Manual of Mental Disorders* (Fifth Edition) (*DSM-5*) clinical diagnosis of bvFTD requires the insidious onset and gradual progression of a neurocognitive disorder combined with at least 3 behavioral symptoms and cognitive decline disproportionately affecting social and/or executive abilities. Behavioral symptoms include (1) disinhibition; (2) apathy or inertia; (3) loss of sympathy or empathy; (4) perseverative, stereotyped, or compulsive/ritualistic behaviors; and (5) hyperorality and dietary changes. The current criteria state that there should be relative sparing of learning and memory and visuospatial (perceptual-motor) function; however, it is now clear that there can be significant impairment in these domains. Symptoms of bvFTD have a striking overlap with those of primary psychiatric disorders.[12] Patients are often first evaluated in general psychiatric settings,[13] and about 50% of patients are initially diagnosed with a primary psychiatric illness.[13] In some cases these were erroneous diagnoses, whereas in others the primary psychiatric disorder is better conceptualized as the prodromal phase of the dementia (eg, psychotic symptoms as the initial manifestation of a *C9ORF72* repeat-expansion genetic mutation[14,15]).

AD classically presents with the insidious progression of cognitive deficits with the predominant deficits in episodic memory.[10] However, atypical presentations of AD are now well recognized in the new diagnostic criteria (McKhann and colleagues,[10] 2011), including logopenic PPA, posterior cortical atrophy (PCA), and dysexecutive or frontal variant AD. These focal presentations of AD are at the extreme end of the spectrum; many patients have multiple domains of cognitive impairment and, thus, would not fulfill the criteria for PPA or PCA but nevertheless do not have a predominantly amnesic presentation. When AD starts before 65 years of age, it is more common for the presentation to be atypical (non-memory), such as apraxia, executive dysfunction, and behavioral symptoms.[16,17]

Although most young-onset dementias are caused by neurodegenerative pathophysiological processes, clinicians must also keep in mind the broad array of pathologies than can present with rapidly progressive dementia.[18] The approach to this problem is reviewed in more detail by Appleby and colleagues, elsewhere in this issue. Among the different causes, paraneoplastic syndromes should be a particular focus of psychiatrists, as some variants (anti–N-methyl-d-aspartate [NMDA], anti-LGI1) can present with predominant, and sometimes isolated, behavioral symptoms.[19,20] In addition, there are multiple other metabolic disturbances and neurologic conditions that can cause or mimic young-onset dementia (**Table 1**).

As previously mentioned, clinical presentations of young-onset dementias often involve a predominance of neuropsychiatric symptoms. Consequently the differential diagnosis includes many primary psychiatric disorders. The overlap between primary psychiatric disorders and dementia is particularly striking for bvFTD. **Table 2** describes both the overlapping and differentiating features between bvFTD and primary psychiatric disorders. Among major differentiating features, in bvFTD, it is unusual for patients to complain of sadness, despair, or anxiety or indeed to acknowledge any suffering or handicap. Patients with bvFTD are generally unlikely to notice and regret functional decline or to show remorse for offensive behavior, whereas patients with primary psychiatric disorders often will (with the exception of those suffering psychosis).[21] FTD and primary psychiatric disorders are not necessarily mutually exclusive, as the latter can be the initial manifestation of a dementia process before obvious cognitive decline.[15,22] Adding a layer of complexity, there is a subgroup of patients meeting the criteria for possible bvFTD who do not show clear deterioration over time and do not have supportive findings on neuroimaging.[23] These bvFTD phenocopies are predominantly men and are less impaired in executive functions, social cognition, and activities of daily living (ADL). Given that the life span is normal and most of the individuals who have come to autopsy did not show frontotemporal lobar degeneration (FTLD) neuropathology, it is generally assumed that these patients do not have a neurodegenerative dementia.[23] However, clinicians need to remain alert, as cases of very slowly progressive FTD secondary to *C9ORF72* have been described.[24]

CLINICAL EXAMINATION
History

The first step when performing a neuropsychiatric assessment of patients suspected of suffering from a young-onset dementia is detailed history taking, with particular attention to the longitudinal progression of symptoms. Starting the interview with open-ended questioning generally allows the physician to identify the most distressing aspects of the illness because patients and families will usually begin with the most pressing or painful parts of the problem. Detailed symptoms should be elicited from patients, including questions related to cognitive decline and functional impairment but also screening for mood, anxiety, sleep, and psychotic disorders. Given the impaired insight associated with some dementias, in particular bvFTD, it is vital to obtain collateral history from a source very familiar with patients, typically a spouse or other close relative. The history is taken not only with respect to the manifest symptoms but also how they deviate from a patient's lifelong temperament, comportment, and habits. Impairments in the different cognitive domains should be explored (attention, working memory, learning and memory, perceptual-motor, language, executive function, social cognition),[25] including more subtle personality changes such as the insidious coarsening of conduct and habits, self-neglect, and the abandonment of work, social routines, and relationships. The informant should be interviewed alone for at least a part of the assessment to facilitate disclosure, as there is often reluctance to describe handicaps and misbehaviors to the patients' hearing. This practice also provides an opportunity to explore the experience of the illness, including the costs and stresses related to the disease.

From a diagnostic perspective, it is essential to capture the chronology of symptoms, noting the approximate onset of the illness, and the timing, order, and progression of the symptoms. In the most common neurodegenerative dementia (AD, FTD), cognitive and behavioral changes start insidiously and progress relatively slowly over months to years. A rapid deterioration over a few weeks to a few months shifts the diagnostic work-up toward a broader differential of rapidly progressing dementias.[18] In bvFTD, changes in conduct, habits, and activity typically precede the development of amnesia, disorientation, or apraxia. The physician should review prior psychiatric history and probe for symptoms and chronologic patterns that may point to a primary psychiatric disorder rather than a neurodegenerative disorder (bvFTD in particular). Lengthy duration of symptoms, lack of progression, and discrete episodes interspersed with a normal state are more suggestive of primary psychiatric disorders. Symptoms that are less suggestive of bvFTD include chronic delusions, hallucinations, long-time episodes of anxiety and depression, longstanding aloofness and awkwardness (spanning decades rather than a few years), recurring mania, depression, or distressing compulsions (compulsions in FTD are generally not accompanied by emotional distress). Although psychotic symptoms are rare in FTD,[26] a notable exception is the striking prevalence of psychosis as the initial presentation of bvFTD secondary to *C9ORF72* mutations.[14,15] In contrast, a behavioral presentation featuring the gradual progression of symptoms, including apathy, loss of empathy, marked personality changes, executive dysfunction, or memory deficits, is suspicious for a young-onset dementia, such as FTD.

The assessment should include a detailed review of neurologic symptoms, such as paresis, abnormal movements, gait imbalance, and falls. These symptoms may point to more uncommon diagnoses (eg, chorea of Huntington disease) or reveal comorbid conditions of neurodegenerative dementias. For example, FTD may be associated with falls and parkinsonian symptoms or with muscle wasting and weakness, suggesting coincident amyotrophic lateral sclerosis (ALS). A general review of system should also be obtained to explore systemic causes (eg, hyperthyroidism, B_{12} deficiency) and rule out unusual adult presentations of lipid storage or mitochondrial diseases that are associated with multiorgan involvement.[27,28]

Family History

A detailed family history of neuropsychiatric disorders should be obtained, as it may provide diagnostic clues and raise the possibility of diseases with autosomal-dominant inheritance patterns. The family history should aim to identify cases of primary psychiatric disorders, early onset dementia, parkinsonism, and ALS. Clinicians should also inquire about poorly defined history of late-onset psychiatric syndromes or unexplained institutionalization in psychiatric hospitals, as these could be

Table 1
Differential diagnosis of young-onset dementia

Category	Disease/Disorder
Traumatic	Traumatic brain injury and postconcussion syndrome Subdural hematoma Chronic traumatic encephalopathy
Infectious	HIV infection and HIV neurocognitive disorder Opportunistic infections Neurosyphilis Viral infections/encephalitides (herpes simplex, CMV, EBV, others) Other infectious encephalitis (bacterial, fungal, parasites) CNS Whipple disease CNS Lyme disease Prion diseases (eg, Creutzfeldt-Jacob disease) Cerebral malaria
Inflammatory/autoimmune	Anti-NMDA encephalitis Anti-LGI1 (anti-VGKC) encephalitis Limbic encephalitis (anti-GAD and others) Systemic lupus erythematous and lupus cerebritis Neurosarcoidosis Hashimoto encephalopathy
Neoplastic	Primary or secondary cerebral neoplasm Paraneoplastic encephalitis (anti-NMDA, anti-Hu, anti-Ma, anti-CRMP5/CV2)
Endocrine/acquired Metabolic	Hepatic encephalopathy Renal failure and uremia Dialysis dementia Hypoglycemia Hypothyroidism/hyperthyroidism Hypothyroidism/hyperparathyroidism Addison disease Cushing disease Wernicke-Korsakoff encephalopathy (thiamine deficiency) Other vitamin deficiencies: B_{12}, folate, niacin, vitamin C, vitamin E Gastric-bypass associated nutritional deficiencies Celiac disease
Vascular	Cerebrovascular accidents (ischemic, hemorrhagic) Vascular dementia CNS vasculitis Transient global amnesia CADASIL Susac syndrome
Neurodegenerative	AD FTD (behavioral variant, primary progressive aphasias) Lewy body dementia Progressive supranuclear palsy Corticobasal degeneration Multiple system atrophy (parkinsonian and cerebellar subtypes) Parkinson disease dementia Huntington disease Idiopathic basal ganglia calcification (Fahr disease) Fragile X-associated tremor/ataxia syndrome

(continued on next page)

Table 1 (continued)	
Category	**Disease/Disorder**
Demyelinating/dysmyelinating	Multiple sclerosis Acute disseminated encephalomyelitis Subacute sclerosing panencephalitis Adrenoleukodystrophy Metachromatic leukodystrophy
Inherited metabolic	Wilson disease Hexosaminidase deficiencies (eg, Tay-Sachs disease, late-onset GM_2 gangliosidosis) Niemann-Pick type C Adult neuronal ceroid-lipofuscinosis (Kufs disease) Neuroacanthocytosis/McLeod syndrome Acute intermittent porphyria Other inborn errors of metabolism (eg, urea cycle defects, MTHFR deficiency, cerebrotendinous xanthomatosis) Mitochondrial disorders MELAS
Psychiatric disorders	Delirium Major depressive disorder Bipolar disorder Schizophrenia Obsessive-compulsive disorder Hoarding disorder Catatonia Attention-deficit/hyperactivity disorder Autism spectrum disorder Personality disorders
Sleep	Obstructive sleep apnea REM sleep behavior disorder
Medications/drugs/toxins	Alcohol (Korsakoff syndrome) Drugs of abuse Heavy metals (eg, lead poisoning) Inhalants Chemotherapy
Other	Cerebral hypoxia Normal pressure hydrocephalus Sagging brain syndrome Ionizing radiation exposure Postradiotherapy cognitive deficits

Abbreviations: CADASIL, cerebral autosomal dominant arteriopathy with subcortical infarcts and leukoencephalopathy; CMV, cytomegalovirus; CNS, central nervous system; EBV, Epstein-Barr virus; HIV, human immunodeficiency virus; MELAS, mitochondrial encephalopathy, lactic acidosis, and strokelike episodes; MTHFR, methylenetetrahydrofolate reductase; REM, rapid eye movement; VGKC, voltage-gated potassium channel.

Adapted from Ducharme S, Murray ED, Price BH. Neuropsychiatric principles and differential diagnosis. In: Stern T, Fava M, Wilens T, et al. editors. Massachusetts General Hospital comprehensive clinical psychiatry. 2nd edition. Philadelphia: Elsevier; 2015; with permission.

caused by young-onset dementia that may not have been specifically diagnosed (eg, Huntington disease, bvFTD). A positive family history of mental illness congruent with behavioral symptoms presented by a patient supports the diagnosis of a primary psychiatric disorder.[29] However, physicians should be aware that a positive family psychiatric history has been shown to bias clinicians toward missing FTD diagnoses.[13]

Table 2
Overlapping and differentiating clinical features of bvFTD and primary psychiatric disorders

Primary Psychiatric Disorders	Overlapping Features with bvFTD	Main Differentiating Features with bvFTD
Major depressive disorder	Lack of interest, decreased motivation, low energy, poor concentration, social and occupational withdrawal	Sustained dysphoria, guilt, and suicidal thoughts in major depression only
Bipolar disorder	Disinhibition, irritability, socially inappropriate behaviors	Euphoria and grandiosity in mania, cyclical nature
Schizophrenia	Low motivation, decreased initiative, social withdrawal, cognitive deficits (executive, working memory)	Psychotic symptoms rare in FTD, different epidemiology (earlier onset in schizophrenia)
Obsessive-compulsive disorder	Identical compulsive behaviors	Lack of obsessions and anxiety in FTD
Hoarding disorder	Pathologic accumulation	Primary hoarding motivated by anxiety and rational for future use as opposed to cognitive disorganization in FTD
Catatonia	Perseveration, stereotypies, mutism, echophenomenon	Fluctuating course, marked acute improvement with benzodiazepines/ECT in catatonia
Autism spectrum disorder	Social cognition impairment	Symptoms present since early childhood without major deterioration over time
ADHD	Distractibility, disorganization, restlessness, impulsive decisions	Symptoms present before 12 years of age, better response to psychostimulants in ADHD
Personality disorders (PD)	Lack of empathy of narcissistic and antisocial PD, impulsivity of borderline PD	Longitudinal maladaptive pattern in PD; problematic behaviors are a break from longitudinal personality in bvFTD

Abbreviations: ADHD, attention-deficit/hyperactivity disorder; ECT, electroconvulsive therapy; PD, personality disorders.

Importantly, any late-onset psychiatric presentation in patients with a family pedigree suspicious for autosomal-dominant dementia should be assessed for the possibility of a neurodegenerative disease. It can be helpful to ask family members to obtain medical records of relatives if possible or to interview distant relatives directly.

Mental Status Examination

All neuropsychiatric assessments of young-onset dementia should include a detailed mental status examination including appearance, attitude and behavior, psychomotor activity, speech, mood, affect, thought process, thought content, perceptions, cognition, insight, and judgment. Attitude and spontaneous behavior during the assessment provide crucial diagnostic information.[21] Patients with bvFTD can be very passive and indifferent to the process or inappropriately disinhibited (eg, repeatedly touching the examiner, offering unrequested marital advice). Diminished comportment (blunted insight, awareness, concern, appropriateness) can suggest a neurodegenerative disease, such as bvFTD. One of the important aspects of the mental status examination is to identify features that are suggestive of a neurodegenerative disease rather than primary psychiatric disorders (see **Table 2**). As an example, the depressed mood and dysphoric affect observed in major depression are usually absent in patients with apathy caused by FTD or other young-onset dementia. The presence of repetitive or compulsive behaviors in the absence of obsessions and anxiety is more compatible with FTD than obsessive-compulsive disorder. The thought process and content also need to be documented. Although patients with young-onset dementia can exhibit tangentiality or confabulation, the presence of disorganization, loosening of associations, and systematized delusions are more suggestive of primary psychotic disorders. The modality and quality of hallucinations also provide diagnostic information (eg, well-formed pleasant visual hallucinations in Lewy Body Dementia (LBD) vs command auditory hallucinations in schizophrenia). The presence and degree of insight into cognitive and behavioral changes gives important clues about the nature of a neurocognitive disorder. Some dementias can be associated with at least partial insight about deficits (vascular, AD), whereas others are almost invariably associated with a complete lack of insight (bvFTD, Huntington disease). Useful instruments to assess and grade the severity of neuropsychiatric symptoms of dementia include the Neuropsychiatric Inventory,[30] the Cambridge Behavioral Inventory,[31] and the Frontal Behavioral Inventory.[32]

Office-Based Cognitive Examination

A cognitive examination can be performed efficiently within the context of a neuropsychiatric consultation and constitutes an essential part of the young-onset dementia assessment. It is informative to start the bedside cognitive examination by quickly assessing attention (forward digit span) and working memory (digit backward, months of the year backward), as this can influence performance in other cognitive domains. Office-based general cognitive testing instruments thought to be more sensitive to young-onset dementia include the Montreal Cognitive Assessment (MoCA)[33] and the Addenbrooke's Cognitive Examination (ACE).[34] The Mini-Mental State Examination (MMSE) is commonly used but lacks sensitivity in the early stages of dementia and does not sufficiently test some cognitive domains, such as executive functions. The Frontal Assessment Battery is a brief (~10 minutes) cognitive and psychomotor assessment that is useful to quickly assess executive functions.[35] Age- and education-adjusted population norms have been determined for these tests.[36,37] It should be noted that some patients in the early stages of FTD achieve normal performance on these cognitive screening tests. Recent studies have suggested that social cognition batteries, including the capacity to recognize facial expression of emotions (Mind in the Eyes test[38]) or identify social norms violations (Faux-Pas test[39]) may be more sensitive than standard cognitive screening tests (ACE, MoCA, MMSE) for the early diagnosis of bvFTD.[40]

In patients suspected of having PPA, clinicians need to spend additional time assessing speech and language. Language components in which deficits can be observed include naming (confrontational naming of objects/pictures), phonemic fluency (list words starting with a letter in 1 minute), semantic fluency (list items from a category in 1 minute), comprehension (perform a 3-step verbal command), paraphasias (spontaneous observation of semantic and phonetic mistakes), grammar and syntax (spontaneous observation and comprehension of irregular noncanonical sentences), and repetition (single word up to multi-words sentences). The pattern of language deficits provides information as to the location of deficits beyond the overly simplistic model of the Broca/Wernicke nonfluent/fluent aphasia (eg, single-object naming impairment caused by left temporal pole atrophy in semantic dementia).

Similarly, a more detailed examination of visuospatial and higher-order visual processing functions is required when there is suspected parieto-occipital involvement (eg, posterior cortical atrophy, LBD, FTD secondary to *GRN* mutations). Bedside tests can include copying 3-dimensional figures (eg, cube in the MoCA); the description of complex images, such as the Cookie Theft Picture for simultagnosia (ie, inability to perceive more than one object at a time); line bisection tasks for hemineglect; and recognition of color/famous faces for agnosia. Limb and buccofacial apraxia should be tested (imitate gesture or pantomime the use of objects such as tools), particularly when there is a suspicion for corticobasal syndrome.[41]

Abnormal results on cognitive tests support the possibility of a young-onset dementia and can serve as a baseline for evaluating changes with passage of time or in response to medication. Depending on availability, a referral for more formal neuropsychological assessment can be very helpful. Although some patients may perform adequately on brief office-based cognitive testing, the neuropsychologist may be able to detect abnormalities on extended testing. Neuropsychological testing also provides scores from standardized tests with well-defined norms that can be followed over time.

Neurologic Examination

The elemental neurologic examination is also an essential component of the neuropsychiatric assessment of young-onset dementia. The goal of the examination is both to identify supportive features of neurodegenerative dementias and to detect signs that would suggest other diagnoses, including cerebrovascular disease, multiple sclerosis, or Parkinson disease (PD). Key elements of the examination include abnormalities in eye movements (restricted vertical gaze in progressive supranuclear palsy), abnormal movements (dyskinesia in Huntington, dystonia in corticobasal syndrome, rest tremor in PD), tone (paratonia, rigidity in PD), primitive reflexes, evidence of motor neuron disease (FTD/ALS), and gait instability (normal pressure hydrocephalus, dementia secondary to alcohol with cerebellar atrophy). Motor Impersistence and distractibility can present challenges during the neurologic examination. Complementary elements of the physical examination including a vascular examination (eg, carotid bruits) should be added depending on the clinical situation. Most patients with AD or FTD will have a normal physical examination in the early stages; or the examination may show only subtle signs suggestive of cerebral dysfunction, such as one or more of snout, sucking, rooting, or grasp reflexes. Subtle signs, such as paratonia and primitive reflexes, are not specific to pathologies or localizable to precise brain areas. Although these findings are compatible with the diagnosis of young-onset dementia, these soft signs have also been found to be prevalent in major psychiatric disorders, such as schizophrenia.[42] Neurologic abnormalities may also emerge as the disease progresses; therefore, the examination should be repeated over time.

DIAGNOSTIC FORMULATION

Once the neuropsychiatric examination is completed, all the information should be integrated to formulate an initial diagnostic impression and investigation plan. The initial task is to classify the patients' overall clinical status within one of the following categories: cognitively normal (with or without subjective cognitive concerns), mild cognitive impairment (*DSM-5* minor neurocognitive disorder), or dementia (*DSM-5* major neurocognitive disorder). Once the overall clinical status is established, the clinical syndrome is described in greater detail (eg, PPA-semantic variant, bvFTD, corticobasal syndrome), including whether or not patients meet *DSM-5* clinical diagnostic criteria. Additional clinical features (eg, with behavioral symptoms or with extrapyra-midal motor signs) or the presence of a secondary diagnosis (eg, with secondary development of motor neuron disease) can be noted. This initial classification allows the clinician to determine the appropriate investigations, including biomarkers. Multi-modal diagnostic tests have two main functions. First, neuroimaging findings can be used to increase the level of confidence in a clinical diagnosis (eg, probable bvFTD if there is supportive imaging markers[43]). Secondly, symptoms, biomarkers, and/or genetic information can be integrated in a probabilistic model to determine the most likely neuropathology underlying the clinical syndrome.

BIOMARKERS

Investigations for young-onset dementias include a combination of basic laboratories, neuroimaging, cerebrospinal fluid (CSF), electrophysiology, and genetic tests. The neuroimaging and genetic tests are covered in more detail by Tighe and colleagues and Goldman, respectively, elsewhere in this issue, but the authors provide an over-view as it pertains to the neuropsychiatric assessment.

Biochemistry and Infectious Serology

As with all initial evaluations of dementia, clinicians should make sure that a basic biochemical panel has been obtained to rule out reversible medical diseases that may be associated with neuropsychiatric symptoms. Tests should minimally include complete blood count, liver and kidney function, electrolytes including calcium levels, thyroid-stimulating hormone, B_{12}/folate, and infectious screening depending on the context (human immunodeficiency virus, syphilis). A more extensive work-up should be performed in rapidly progressing dementia cases (reviewed elsewhere this issue by Appleby and colleagues).

Neuroimaging

Neuroimaging is probably the most crucial part of the diagnostic work-up of young-onset dementia, both to identify regional patterns of atrophy supportive of specific de-mentia subtypes (eg, left temporal pole atrophy in semantic PPA) and to rule out different pathophysiological processes, such as strokes, tumors, normal pressure hy-drocephalus, sagging brain syndrome,[44] cerebral autosomal-dominant arteriopathy with subcortical infarcts and leukoencephalopathy, and various white matter diseases (see **Table 1**). Both structural (preferably MRI) and functional (PET, single-photon emission computed tomography) neuroimaging may be valuable for the Investigation of anatomic, metabolic, or perfusion abnormalities in neurodegenerative dementias. It should be noted that, in some FTD cases, both structural and functional neuroimaging may be normal early in the course of the disease.[45]

With the advent of neuroimaging tracers that bind to specific pathologic molecules, such as Pittsburgh compound B[46] for amyloid or the growing number of putative tau ligands,[47–50] it is now becoming possible to investigate molecular diagnoses in vivo. These tests are currently used in research or by specialized memory clinics. Efforts are underway to validate these markers for clinical use and develop additional tracers for specific pathologic processes.

Cerebrospinal Fluid

CSF analysis is an essential investigation to rule out infectious, inflammatory, or neoplastic disorders in patients with atypical features or a more rapid course.[18] Quan-tification of Aβ-42 amyloid (decreased), phosphorylated-tau (elevated), and total tau (elevated) is now becoming more available as a biomarker of AD and can often be very valuable in the assessment of young patients with dementia.[51,52] One study using data from the Alzheimer's Disease Neuroimaging Initiative found that the combination of Aβ-42 and total tau has a positive predictive value of 85.7% and a negative predictive value of 84.6% for autopsy-proven cases of AD.[53] CSF biomarkers are also being investigated in FTLD,[54] but results are not consistent enough for use in clinical practice.

Electrophysiology

An electroencephalography (EEG) can be a useful screening tool for encephalopathy in cases of rapidly progressing dementias or when epileptic activity is suspected (eg, non-convulsive status). An EEG is not commonly recommended in the diagnostic evaluation of neurodegenerative dementias but may show diffuse slowing in more advanced cases. EEG is usually normal in the early stages of FTD but may demonstrate anterior or focal slowing consistent with frontal neurodegeneration as the disease progresses.

If motor neuron disease is suspected based on clinical examination (eg, fasciculation, muscle weakness with atrophy, dysphagia, slurred speech), an electromyography should be obtained to determine the presence of upper or lower motor neuron dysfunction. This test can provide important prognostic information given that the FTD/ALS complex tends to progress faster than isolated FTD.[55]

Genetic Studies

Autosomal-dominant mutations have been associated with AD (PS1, PS2, APP), FTD (GRN, MAPT, C9ORF72), Huntington disease (huntingtin CAG repeat), Fahr disease (SLC20A2), and others. There are also various autosomal-recessive conditions that can present with cognitive decline (see Table 1). The genetic aspects of young-onset dementia are reviewed in more detail elsewhere in this issue by Goldman. In summary, clinicians should obtain a detailed family history to determine the possibility of a causal genetic mutation in patients with neurodegenerative diseases. Risk stratifications have been developed for this purpose in FTLD.[56] In cases when a genetic cause is suspected, the authors recommend a genetic consultation for counseling before testing for mutations.

PSYCHOSOCIAL ASPECTS

In parallel to the diagnostic assessment, the neuropsychiatric evaluation should include a careful documentation of disabilities, as it constitutes the basis for planning immediate and future care. These disabilities include handicaps, such as disorientation to situations, impaired communication, decline in self-care, abnormal feeding, and loss of bladder, and bowel control. Using instruments designed to quantify disability can facilitate this process.[57]

The management of patients with young-onset dementia generally requires the expertise of an experienced multidisciplinary team.[58,59] The neuropsychiatric evaluation should serve to identify specific needs for individual patients. These needs may include speech and language therapy for communication or swallowing issues, occupational therapy for problems with hand-eye coordination or planning that impacts ADLs, physical therapy for gait disorders, social work assistance with disability compensation, and in some cases psychotherapy (for patients and/or families). A driving assessment and determination of financial and health care competency are critical components. Early on in the evaluation process, health care providers should dedicate time to provide specialized education to patients/families, including referral to the Association for FTD (http://www.theaftd.org/) and the Alzheimer's Association (http://www.alz.org).

LONGITUDINAL ASSESSMENT

Despite investigations, diagnostic ambiguity can persist for prolonged periods after the initial neuropsychiatric evaluation. This ambiguity is particularly common in predominantly behavioral presentations in which the differential diagnosis is between bvFTD, nonprogressive bvFTD, and primary psychiatric disorders. In the authors' opinion, these diagnostic uncertainties should be honestly shared with patients and caregivers. It is crucial to provide longitudinal follow-up, as this period of uncertainty can be quite distressing. The authors' approach is to repeat a thorough assessment with cognitive testing and imaging on a yearly basis until the final diagnosis is established. Once a diagnosis of young-onset dementia is confirmed, it is important to provide ongoing monitoring and care through the course of the illness or to refer patients to a specialty center. In the authors' practice, they always discuss the value of autopsy with the families and with the patients if possible. Indeed, despite continued improvements in the use of clinical and biomarker data for probabilistic prediction of pathology, every specialized center continues to observe surprising cases.

SUMMARY

Identifying and diagnosing young-onset dementia is a complex neuropsychiatric challenge, as these patients often present with predominant behavioral features and are outside of the typical demographic for dementia. Psychiatrists have a crucial role in recognizing cases of young-onset dementias, initiating investigations, and referring patients to specialized neurocognitive clinics. This article attempts to provide a framework for the initial neuropsychiatric evaluation of these patients. Although there are, unfortunately, no current curative treatments for neurodegenerative dementias, various medications can reduce neuropsychiatric symptoms, such as agitation and psychosis, thereby ameliorating the suffering of patients and caretakers. In addition, making an accurate and rapid diagnosis is a necessary step for patients and their family to adequately prepare for the inexorable progression of these neurodegenerative diseases. Finally, once a diagnosis of young-onset dementia is confirmed, clinicians have the responsibility to guide patients and relatives through the appropriate resources (eg, day programs, nursing homes, end-of-life care) as the disease evolves in order to minimize psychosocial complications.

REFERENCES

1. McMurtray A, Clark DG, Christine D, et al. Early-onset dementia: frequency and causes compared to late-onset dementia. Dement Geriatr Cogn Disord 2006;21: 59–64.
2. Shinagawa S, Ikeda M, Toyota Y, et al. Frequency and clinical characteristics of early-onset dementia in consecutive patients in a memory clinic. Demont Goriatr Cogn Disord 2007;24:42–7.
3. Picard C, Pasquier F, Martinaud O, et al. Early onset dementia: characteristics in a large cohort from academic memory clinics. Alzheimer Dis Assoc Disord 2011; 25:203–5.
4. Garre-Olmo J, Batlle DG, del Mar Fernandez M, et al. Incidence and subtypes of early-onset dementia in a geographically defined general population. Neurology 2010;75:1249–55.

5. Lambert MA, Bickel H, Prince M, et al. Estimating the burden of early onset dementia; systematic review of disease prevalence. Eur J Neurol 2014;21:563–9.
6. Mendez MF. The accurate diagnosis of early-onset dementia. Int J Psychiatry Med 2006;36:401–12.
7. Alladi S, Xuereb J, Bak T, et al. Focal cortical presentations of Alzheimer's disease. Brain 2007;130:2636–45.
8. Rademakers R, Neumann M, Mackenzie IR. Advances in understanding the molecular basis of frontotemporal dementia. Nat Rev Neurol 2012;8:423–34.
9. Rascovsky K, Hodges JR, Knopman D, et al. Sensitivity of revised diagnostic criteria for the behavioural variant of frontotemporal dementia. Brain 2011;134: 2456–77.
10. McKhann G, Knopman D, Chertkow H, et al. The diagnosis of dementia due to Alzheimer's disease: recommendations from the National Institute on Aging - Alzheimer's Association workgroups on diagnostic guidelines for Alzheimer's disease. Alzheimers Dement 2011;7:263–9.
11. Onyike CU, Diehl-Schmid J. The epidemiology of frontotemporal dementia. Int Rev Psychiatry 2013;25:130–7.
12. Pose M, Cetkovich M, Gleichgerrcht E, et al. The overlap of symptomatic dimensions between frontotemporal dementia and several psychiatric disorders that appear in late adulthood. Int Rev Psychiatry 2013;25:159–67.
13. Woolley JD, Khan BK, Murthy NK, et al. The diagnostic challenge of psychiatric symptoms in neurodegenerative disease; rates of and risk factors for prior psychiatric diagnosis in patients with early neurodegenerative disease. J Clin Psychiatry 2011;72:126.
14. Snowden JS, Rollinson S, Thompson JC, et al. Distinct clinical and pathological characteristics of frontotemporal dementia associated with C9ORF72 mutations. Brain 2012;135:693–708.
15. Galimberti D, Fenoglio C, Serpente M, et al. Autosomal dominant frontotemporal lobar degeneration due to the C9ORF72 hexanucleotide repeat expansion: late-onset psychotic clinical presentation. Biol Psychiatry 2013;74:384–91.
16. Koedam EL, Lauffer V, van der Vlies AE, et al. Early-versus late-onset Alzheimer's disease: more than age alone. J Alzheimers Dis 2010;19:1401–8.
17. Balasa M, Gelpi E, Antonell A, et al. Clinical features and APOE genotype of pathologically proven early-onset Alzheimer disease. Neurology 2011;76:1720–5.
18. Paterson RW, Takada LT, Geschwind MD. Diagnosis and treatment of rapidly progressive dementias. Neurol Clin Pract 2012;2:187–200.
19. Kayser MS, Kohler CG, Dalmau J. Psychiatric manifestations of paraneoplastic disorders. Am J Psychiatry 2010;167:1039–50.
20. Kayser MS, Titulaer MJ, Gresa-Arribas N, et al. Frequency and characteristics of isolated psychiatric episodes in anti–N-methyl-d-aspartate receptor encephalitis. JAMA Neurol 2013;70:1133–9.
21. Rankin KP, Santos-Modesitt W, Kramer JH, et al. Spontaneous social behaviors discriminate behavioral dementias from psychiatric disorders and other dementias. J Clin Psychiatry 2008;69:60–73.
22. Floris G, Borghero G, Cannas A, et al. Bipolar affective disorder preceding frontotemporal dementia in a patient with C9ORF72 mutation: is there a genetic link between these two disorders? J Neurol 2013;260:1155–7.
23. Kipps CM, Hodges JR, Hornberger M. Nonprogressive behavioural frontotemporal dementia: recent developments and clinical implications of the 'bvFTD phenocopy syndrome'. Curr Opin Neurol 2010;23:628–32.

24. Khan BK, Yokoyama JS, Takada LT, et al. Atypical, slowly progressive behavioural variant frontotemporal dementia associated with C9ORF72 hexanucleotide expansion. J Neurol Neurosurg Psychiatry 2012;83:358–64.
25. American Psychiatric Association. Diagnostic and statistical manual of mental disorders. 5th edition. Arlington (VA): American Psychiatric Association; 2013.
26. Mendez MF, Shapira JS, Woods RJ, et al. Psychotic symptoms in frontotemporal dementia: prevalence and review. Dement Geriatr Cogn Disord 2008;25:206–11.
27. Anglin RE, Tarnopolsky MA, Mazurek MF, et al. The psychiatric presentation of mitochondrial disorders in adults. J Neuropsychiatry Clin Neurosci 2012;24: 394–409.
28. Sedel F, Baumann N, Turpin JC, et al. Psychiatric manifestations revealing inborn errors of metabolism in adolescents and adults. J Inherit Metab Dis 2007;30: 631–41.
29. Panegyres PK, Graves A, Frencham KA. The clinical differentiation of fronto-temporal dementia from psychiatric disease. Neuropsychiatr Dis Treat 2007;3:637.
30. Cummings JL, Mega M, Gray K, et al. The neuropsychiatric inventory: comprehensive assessment of psychopathology in dementia. Neurology 1994;44:2308.
31. Wear HJ, Wedderburn CJ, Mioshi E, et al. The Cambridge behavioural inventory revised. Dement Neuropsychol 2008;2:102–7.
32. Kertesz A, Davidson W, Fox H. Frontal behavioral inventory: diagnostic criteria for frontal lobe dementia. Can J Neurol Sci 1997;24:29–36.
33. Nasreddine ZS, Phillips NA, Bédirian V, et al. The Montreal Cognitive Assessment, MoCA: a brief screening tool for mild cognitive impairment. J Am Geriatr Soc 2005;53:695–9.
34. Mathuranath PS, Nestor PJ, Berrios GE, et al. A brief cognitive test battery to differentiate Alzheimer's disease and frontotemporal dementia. Neurology 2000; 55:1613–20.
35. Dubois B, Slachevsky A, Litvan I, et al. The FAB: a frontal assessment battery at bedside. Neurology 2000;55:1621–6.
36. Rossetti HC, Lacritz LH, Cullum CM, et al. Normative data for the Montreal Cognitive Assessment (MoCA) in a population-based sample. Neurology 2011;77: 1272–5.
37. Appollonio I, Leone M, Isella V, et al. The Frontal Assessment Battery (FAB): normative values in an Italian population sample. Neurol Sci 2005;26:108–16.
38. Baron-Cohen S, Wheelwright S, Hill J, et al. The "Reading the mind in the eyes" test revised version: a study with normal adults, and adults with Asperger syndrome or high-functioning autism. J Child Psychol Psychiatry 2001;42:241–51.
39. Baron-Cohen S, O'Riordan M, Stone V, et al. Recognition of faux pas by normally developing children and children with Asperger syndrome or high-functioning autism. J Autism Dev Disord 1999;29:407–18.
40. Torralva T, Roca M, Gleichgerrcht E, et al. A neuropsychological battery to detect specific executive and social cognitive impairments in early frontotemporal dementia. Brain 2009;132:1299–309.
41. Armstrong MJ, Litvan I, Lang AE, et al. Criteria for the diagnosis of corticobasal degeneration. Neurology 2013;80:496–503.
42. Chan RC, Xu T, Heinrichs RW, et al. Neurological soft signs in schizophrenia: a meta-analysis. Schizophr Bull 2010;36:1089–104.
43. Harris JM, Gall C, Thompson JC, et al. Sensitivity and specificity of FTDC criteria for behavioral variant frontotemporal dementia. Neurology 2013;80:1881–7.

44. Wicklund M, Mokri B, Drubach D, et al. Frontotemporal brain sagging syndrome: an SIH-like presentation mimicking FTD. Neurology 2011;76:1377–82.

45. Gregory CA, Serra-Mestres J, Hodges JR. Early diagnosis of the frontal variant of frontotemporal dementia: how sensitive are standard neuroimaging and neuropsychologic tests? Neuropsychiatry Neuropsychol Behav Neurol 1999;12: 128–35.

46. Klunk WE, Engler H, Nordberg A, et al. Imaging brain amyloid in Alzheimer's disease with Pittsburgh compound-B. Ann Neurol 2004;55:306–19.

47. Small GW, Kepe V, Ercoli LM, et al. PET of brain amyloid and tau in mild cognitive impairment. N Engl J Med 2006;355:2652–63.

48. Chien DT, Bahri S, Szardenings AK, et al. Early clinical PET imaging results with the novel PHF-tau radioligand [F-18]-T807. J Alzheimers Dis 2013;34:457–68.

49. Maruyama M, Shimada H, Suhara T, et al. Imaging of tau pathology in a tauopathy mouse model and in Alzheimer patients compared to normal controls. Neuron 2013;79:1094–108.

50. Fodero-Tavoletti MT, Okamura N, Furumoto S, et al. 18F-THK523: a novel in vivo tau imaging ligand for Alzheimer's disease. Brain 2011;134:1089–100.

51. Blennow K, Hampel H, Weiner M, et al. Cerebrospinal fluid and plasma biomarkers in Alzheimer disease. Nat Rev Neurol 2010;6:131–44.

52. Tapiola T, Alafuzoff I, Herukka SK, et al. Cerebrospinal fluid β-amyloid 42 and tau proteins as biomarkers of Alzheimer-type pathologic changes in the brain. JAMA Neurol 2009;66:382–9.

53. Shaw LM, Vanderstichele H, Knapik-Czajka M, et al. Cerebrospinal fluid biomarker signature in Alzheimer's disease neuroimaging initiative subjects. Ann Neurol 2009;65:403–13.

54. Hu WT, Chen-Plotkin A, Grossman M, et al. Novel CSF biomarkers for frontotemporal lobar degenerations. Neurology 2011;75:2079–86.

55. Hodges J, Davies R, Xuereb J, et al. Survival in frontotemporal dementia. Neurology 2003;61:349–54.

56. Wood EM, Falcone D, Suh E, et al. Development and validation of pedigree classification criteria for frontotemporal lobar degeneration. JAMA Neurol 2013; 70(11):1411–7.

57. Onyike CU, Sloane KL, Smyth SF, et al. Estimating severity of illness and disability in frontotemporal dementia: preliminary analysis of the Dementia Disability Rating (DDR). Acta Neuropsychol 2011;9:141–53.

58. Gitlin LN, Kales HC, Lyketsos CG. Nonpharmacologic management of behavioral symptoms in dementia. JAMA 2012;308:2020–9.

59. Shnall A, Agate A, Grinberg A, et al. Development of supportive services for frontotemporal dementias through community engagement. Int Rev Psychiatry 2013; 25:246–52.

Neuropsychological Assessment and Differential Diagnosis in Young-Onset Dementias

Emilia J. Sitek, PhD[a,b], Anna Barczak, PhD[c],
Michał Harciarek, PhD[d,*]

KEYWORDS

- Alzheimer's disease • Frontotemporal dementia • Primary progressive aphasia
- Progressive supranuclear palsy • Posterior cortical atrophy

KEY POINTS

- Most young-onset dementia syndromes belong to the spectrum of early-onset Alzheimer's disease or frontotemporal dementia.
- Patients with young-onset dementia usually present with early behavior, executive, or language changes.
- Episodic memory impairment is rarely seen at onset.
- Comprehensive neuropsychological assessment is crucial to the young-onset dementia diagnosis.

YOUNG-ONSET DEMENTIAS—THE ROLE OF NEUROPSYCHOLOGY

Young-onset dementias (YODs) are a heterogeneous group of disorders comprising mainly early-onset adult primary neurodegenerative diseases (in contrast to late onset), late-onset forms of childhood neurodegenerative conditions (eg, mitochondrial disorders), vascular dementia (VaD), various dementia syndromes with potentially reversible etiologies (eg, autoimmune, infectious diseases), and dementias related to substance abuse. The diagnosis of YOD is usually based on history (with the crucial

The authors have nothing to disclose.
[a] Neurology Department, St. Adalbert Hospital, Copernicus PL Sp. z o.o., Al. Jana Pawła II 50, Gdansk 80-462, Poland; [b] Neurological and Psychiatric Nursing Department, Medical University of Gdansk, Al. Jana Pawła II 50, Gdansk 80-462, Poland; [c] Neurodegenerative Department, Neurology Clinic, MSW Hospital, Wołoska 137, Warsaw 02-507, Poland; [d] Clinical Psychology and Neuropsychology Unit, Institute of Psychology, University of Gdansk, Bażyńskiego 4, Gdansk 80-952, Poland
* Corresponding author.
E-mail address: psymh@ug.edu.pl

Psychiatr Clin N Am 38 (2015) 265–279
http://dx.doi.org/10.1016/j.psc.2015.01.003
0193-953X/15/$ – see front matter © 2015 Elsevier Inc. All rights reserved.

Abbreviations	
ACE-III	Addenbrooke's Cognitive Examination-III
AD	Alzheimer's disease
bvFTD	Behavioral variant of frontotemporal dementia
CBS	Corticobasal syndrome
DLB	Dementia with Lewy bodies
DRS-2	Mattis Dementia Rating Scale-2
ECAS	Edinburgh Cognitive and Behavioral ALS Screen
EOAD	Early-onset Alzheimer's disease
FTD	Frontotemporal dementia
HD	Huntington's disease
lvPPA	Logopenic variant of primary progressive aphasia
MMSE	Mini-Mental State Examination
nfvPPA	Nonfluent variant of primary progressive aphasia
PCA	Posterior cortical atrophy
PPA	Primary progressive aphasia
PSP	Progressive supranuclear palsy
svPPA	Semantic variant of primary progressive aphasia
VaD	Vascular dementia
VOSP	Visual Object and Space Perception Battery
YOAD	Young-onset Alzheimer's disease (also known as EOAD, early-onset AD)
YOD	Young-onset dementia

input from the informant), neuropsychiatric, cognitive and motor examination, neuro-imaging, and laboratory findings, although for some diseases, genetic testing is becoming increasingly useful in the clinical practice.[1] The diagnosis of other disorders, such as normal-pressure hydrocephalus or mitochondrial disorder, is based mainly on physical, imaging, and laboratory findings. Thus, in this review, these disorders are not discussed in detail.

Neuropsychological assessment in YOD may serve several purposes:

1. Differentiating subjective cognitive complaints from cognitive impairment
2. Determining the presence and severity of cognitive impairment
3. Determining the impact of emotional factors (eg, anxiety, depressed mood) on cognitive performance
4. Determining the patient's cognitive profile to contribute to the differential diagnosis of dementia

Aims 1 through 3 have been extensively discussed in the literature[2] and exceed the scope of this review, which focuses on the role of neuropsychology in delineating the patient's cognitive profile. It is well documented that the integration of prospective clinical and neuropsychological data (eg, "anterior" vs "posterior" cognitive profile) associated with time course of illness is highly predictive of pathology on autopsy examination.[3]

For the sake of brevity, some specific aspects of neuropsychological examination, such as the assessment of reading, writing and calculation, were omitted in this review.

NEUROPSYCHOLOGICAL SCREENING ASSESSMENT IN YOUNG-ONSET DEMENTIA

Because YOD refers to individuals younger than 65, the cognitive screening tools aimed at this population need to be more sensitive to subtle cognitive alterations than coarse-grained measures, such as Mini-Mental State Examination (MMSE).[4]

Addenbrooke's Cognitive Examination-III (ACE-III),[5] Mattis Dementia Rating Scale-2 (DRS-2),[6] and Edinburgh Cognitive and Behavioral ALS Screen (ECAS)[7] are not only more sensitive to cognitive impairment than MMSE, but they also help to generate hypotheses about the patient's cognitive profile (**Table 1**).[8] Most of the available cognitive screeners, designed to detect Alzheimer's disease (AD), focus on episodic memory assessment. In contrast, ACE-III (with a strong language focus) and DRS-2 (addressing more thoroughly executive function) prove useful in the differential diagnosis of dementias, as in the case of atypical Parkinsonian syndromes.[9] However, none of these comprehensive screeners covers the range of cognitive functions (see **Table 1**), including various aspects of executive function, hemispatial neglect, or praxis. The Oxford Cognitive Screen, a short version of Birmingham Cognitive Screen (aimed mainly at stroke patients),[10] permits the assessment of hemispatial neglect. Also, few specific screeners for the assessment of executive function were created, such as Frontal Assessment Battery[11] and INECO Frontal Screening.[12] In many cases only a full neuropsychological assessment may provide a valid and comprehensive cognitive profile, allowing for a reliable diagnosis.

RATIONALE FOR COMPREHENSIVE NEUROPSYCHOLOGICAL ASSESSMENT

Comprehensive neuropsychological assessment is crucial in the differential diagnosis of some YOD, especially those with underlying neurodegenerative conditions. Although this report focuses mainly on early-onset neurodegenerative diseases, such highly prevalent conditions such as VaD and dementia related to substance abuse are also discussed. In this review, cognitive profiles of various YOD syndromes are compared against late-onset AD, as it remains the recognized dementia.

The order in which neuropsychological tests are given and their interpretation are usually dictated by the multifactorial nature of cognitive measures.[13] None of the cognitive domains should be tested in isolation, and the performance on a neuropsychological tests addressing a specific cognitive domain typically depends on other cognitive processes (eg, card sorting tasks aimed at measuring executive function also require good visual perception). Although some deficits become apparent only during direct testing, language and executive impairments may lead to impaired scores throughout the testing session, as instruction comprehension and focused cooperation are crucial for valid performance. Because most of the test instructions are given in a verbal format, assessing language (speech comprehension in particular) is a prerequisite for further testing. Thus, verbal and visual memory assessment should be preceded by language and visuospatial function examination, respectively. Further, both verbal and visual impairments may lead to failure on praxis and executive tasks. Moreover, to avoid misinterpretation of the results, executive function is directly tested only after all other cognitive domains are already covered (**Fig. 1**).

HOW TO OPTIMIZE NEUROPSYCHOLOGICAL ASSESSMENT

Full neuropsychological assessment may be lengthy and tiring for the patient. Thus, to allow sufficient focus on predominant deficits, the patient's background information, cognitive and neuropsychiatric history, neurologic assessment data, and neuroimaging results should be available for the neuropsychologist before commencing the assessment. Thanks to generating individual hypotheses, the testing time may be reduced, more attention may be given to predominant areas of interest, and the patient's frustration may be kept to a minimum, for example, if corticobasal syndrome (CBS) is suspected, a more detailed assessment of domains that are sometimes

Table 1
Comparison of clinical utility of ACE-III, ECAS, DRS-2, and MMSE

Feature	ACE-III	ECAS	DRS-2	MMSE
			Test	
Administration time[a]	15–30 min	15–30 min	15–45 min	5–10 min
Cost	Free available online	Free available online	Examination booklet and scoring sheets need to be purchased	Currently scoring sheets need to be purchased
Alternate versions	Yes	No	Yes	No
Language versions	Many language adaptations	No	Few	Many language adaptations
Training	2-part training available online	Training materials available online	No	No
Language dependent	+++	++	+	+++
Motor dependent	++	No	+	+
Attention/working memory	1 task (serial 7s)	Spelling, reverse digit span	Attention items focus on either speech comprehension or visual search	1 task (serial 7s)
Visuospatial functions	5 tasks assessing object perception, space perception, and construction	3 tasks assessing space perception	Few relatively easy items assessing construction	1 item addressing construction
Language functions	Quite comprehensive assessment: naming, verbal fluency, speech comprehension, repetition, reading writing	Naming, verbal fluency; spelling	No specific language tasks; speech comprehension, repetition, reading + verbal fluency	Relatively easy language items
Semantic memory	Verbal and verbal-visual semantics	Verbal-visual semantics	No	No
Abstract thinking	No	No	Verbal and nonverbal task	No
Episodic memory	Learning task with 3 trials, delayed recall & recognition, ecologically valid; 3-word recall after distraction	Story recall (immediate & delayed) and recognition	Few tasks based only on recall, few other tasks on recognition (verbal and visual)	3-word recall after distraction
Executive function	Only verbal fluency	Verbal fluency; alternating task; sentence completion requiring inhibition (inspired by Hayling test)	Subscale addressing initiation and perseveration	No
Theory of mind	No	Yes	No	No

"+" refers to the extent/degree of dependence.
[a] Based on authors' clinical experience.

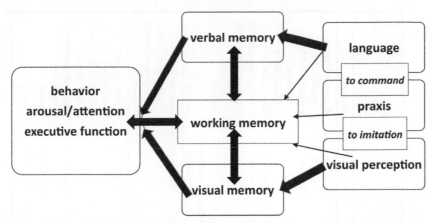

Fig. 1. Neuropsychological assessment in YOD—overview of main cognitive domains.

overlooked, such as visual versus tactile neglect, apraxia profile, or cortical discrimination, would be beneficial.

BEHAVIOR ASSESSMENT

Behavioral and psychological symptoms of dementia represent the spectrum of noncognitive symptoms that may be seen in YOD. The assessment of these symptoms is essential for the diagnosis and treatment of YOD, as neuropsychiatric features of dementia are the core or supportive diagnostic traits of most YODs, as they are often very specific.[14] Behavioral and psychological symptoms of dementia include disinhibition, loss of empathy, apathy, stereotyped/ritualistic habits, impulsivity or challenging behaviors, psychotic symptoms, changes in eating habits (stereotyped or especially craving of sweet foods), sleep pattern, and sexual behavior abnormalities **(Table 2)**.[15] In YOD, behavioral disturbances can herald cognitive impairment (eg, a variety of psychiatric symptoms in Huntington's disease [HD] or apathy or impulsivity in progressive supranuclear palsy [PSP]), can predominate clinical manifestation (eg, in behavioral variant of frontotemporal dementia [bvFTD]),[16] or simply coexist with cognitive decline (apathy in PSP). These behavioral disturbances vary in different types of YOD, however, increase as the disease advances.[17] If neuropsychiatric examination was not performed before neuropsychological assessment, the neuropsychologist needs to address behavioral symptoms in the interview with a patient and especially his or her proxy, as the neuropsychiatric profile is important for planning the assessment and the interpretation of the results of cognitive examination.

The observation of a patient during testing should address many aspects of behavior, such as, overall rate of performance, latency to provide the answers, cognitive insight into difficulties, emotional reactions to failure, ability to initiate activities and switch from one activity to another, intrusions from previous tasks, or perseverative tendencies. Recognition of qualitative characteristics of performance throughout testing may sometimes be more helpful in the process of differential diagnosis than the test scores.[18,19]

LANGUAGE ASSESSMENT

Comprehensive language examination should encompass spontaneous and narrative speech assessment, word finding (both in speech and on confrontation naming),

Table 2
Cognitive profile of different YOD syndromes at presentation

Dementia Type	Variant	Function					
		Behavior	Executive & Attention	Language	Visuospatial	Praxis	Memory
AD	Amnestic	Irritability/mild depression	Mildly impaired	Anomia	Mildly impaired	May be impaired	**Amnestic memory profile**
	Language (lvPPA)	Normal	Typically spared	**Impaired phonology**	Spared	Spared	**Verbal short-term memory impairment**
	Executive variant	**Disinhibition**	Impaired	Reduced speech output	Spared	Typically spared	Cued recall & recognition better than spontaneous recall
	Visual (PCA)	Normal	Impaired visual attention	Spared	**Impaired object/space perception**	Spatially impaired	Spared
	Apraxic variant	Typically spared	Impaired	Spared	Spared	**Impaired**	Spared
VaD	Pure or mixed with AD	Irritability & apathy	**Poor initiation; working memory impairment**	Possible anomia	Usually impaired construction	Usually spared	Cued recall & recognition better than spontaneous recall
	CADASIL	Apathy					
FTD	Behavioral variant	**Pronounced disinhibition and indifference**	Often impaired from onset	Reduced speech output	Spared	Spared	Relatively well preserved, retrieval problems may appear
	svPPA/Semantic dementia	Cravings, food fads	Initially spared	**Anomia; impaired semantics**	Spared	Spared	**Impaired semantic memory**
	nfvPPA	Mild depression	Initially spared	**Agrammatism/ apraxia of speech/ effortful speech**	Spared	Usually impaired	Spared

CBS	Apathy	Mild deficits	Possible apraxia of speech/nonfluency	Unilateral neglect in some cases; perception better than construction	**Impaired**	Cued recall & recognition better than spontaneous recall
PSP	Apathy/ disinhibition, impulsivity	**Perseveration, poor inhibition**	Possible nonfluency/ apraxia of speech	Relatively well preserved	Usually spared	Cued recall & recognition better than spontaneous recall
HD	Variety of neuropsychiatric manifestations	**Impaired**	Reduced spontaneous speech	Mildly impaired	Relatively preserved	Cued recall & recognition better than spontaneous recall
Parkinson's disease with dementia/DLB	Apathy	**Impaired**	Anomia	Impaired	Relatively preserved	Cued recall & recognition better than spontaneous recall
Alcohol related	Irritability, mood lability	Impaired cognitive control	Mildly affected	Mildly affected	Preserved	**Predominant amnesic memory profile**

Predominant deficit for each syndrome is presented in bold.

Abbreviation: CADASIL, Cerebral Autosomal-Dominant Arteriopathy with Subcortical Infarcts and Leukoencephalopathy.

comprehension (on word level and sentence level in terms of length and syntactic complexity) and repetition (of words and sentences) (**Fig. 2**). Whenever possible, reading, writing, and calculation should also be assessed, as it may provide clues to the patient's cognitive profile.

Nonfluent/agrammatic speech with difficulty forming sentences and apraxia of speech are hallmarks of the nonfluent variant of primary progressive aphasia (nfvPPA).[20,21] However, such problems may also appear in the course of CBS and PSP.[22] Losing track in conversation is typical for AD and VaD. Moreover, patients with bvFTD, despite well-preserved phonology, syntax, and semantics, often present with reduced spontaneous speech output.[23]

Although word-finding difficulties and anomia basically occur in every dementia syndrome, prominent word-finding impairment characterizes primary progressive aphasias (PPA), particularly the logopenic variant of PPA (lvPPA) (often referred to as the language variant of AD) and the semantic variant of PPA (svPPA).[20,21] In AD, word comprehension is much better preserved than word finding, whereas in svPPA these processes are usually equally impaired, as they result from a conceptual rather than purely verbal deficit (see later discussion). Deficient verbal fluency (especially phonemic) in the context of much better preserved naming is usually attributed to executive failure in searching through a mental lexicon. Such a pattern is typical for bvFTD and syndromes with frontostriatal involvement (eg, HD and PSP).[24] Poor confrontation naming may stem not only from word-finding problems but also from perceptual difficulties (eg, in posterior cortical atrophy [PCA] or dementia with Lewy bodies [DLB]—failure to form a correct percept) or semantic impairment (in svPPA—failure to attribute meaning to the percept). These problems may be differentiated through a verbal description task or generation of definitions (typically impaired in svPPA and may be much better preserved than confrontation naming in PCA or DLB) and copying line drawing (intact in svPPA and deficient in PCA).[15]

Patterns of sentence comprehension and repetition are particularly useful in the differential diagnosis of nfvPPA and lvPPA. Patients with lvPPA have difficulties repeating and understanding long sentences owing to defective phonologic processing, whereas individuals with nfvPPA struggle more with repeating phonologically complex

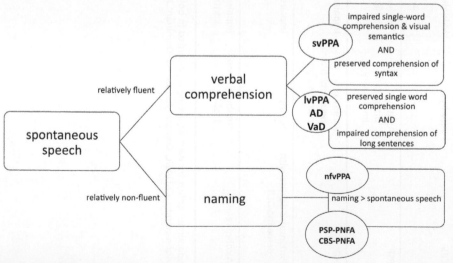

Fig. 2. Language assessment.

words and syllable strings. In nfvPPA, syntax comprehension is more challenging than sentence length.[20,21]

VISUOSPATIAL ASSESSMENT

Visuospatial assessment in the context of suspected dementia typically encompasses object perception, spatial perception, construction, and visual search (**Fig. 3**). Subtests from the Visual Object and Space Perception Battery (VOSP)[25] are particularly useful for differentiating object (eg, incomplete letters) and space perception (eg, cube analysis). Visual search can be assessed through cancellation tasks or Trail Making Test A.[13]

Prominent object perception deficits affecting object recognition are suggestive of PCA.[26] However, mild problems with object recognition may also appear in DLB, AD, and VaD. If a patient is not able to recognize the identity of the contour drawing but is able to copy it, the problem is likely to be semantic.[15] Face recognition tasks may be used in the diagnosis of right temporal variant of frontotemporal lobar degeneration in which prosopagnosia may be the first clinical features.[27] Assessment of visuospatial function in CBS can predict AD or non-AD pathology; for example, low performance on cube analysis from VOSP is suggestive of underlying AD pathologic condition in CBS.[28]

Impaired construction in the context of good visuoperceptual function raises the query of executive problems (impulsive and perseverative errors lead to disorganized drawing,[19] frequently observed in bvFTD or PSP) or apraxia (resulting in distorted spatial relationships, especially in 3 dimensions, eg, in CBS).

Unilateral neglect rarely occurs in YOD. It may appear in CBS and VaD, and there may be some asymmetry in PCA as well. If CBS is suspected, it is worth testing for visual and sensory extinction, cortical sensory loss, and number processing.[29]

PRAXIS ASSESSMENT

The major 4 types of apraxia are limb-kinetic, ideomotor, ideational or conceptual, and oral (buccofacial). Assessment aimed at the first 3 apraxia syndromes (limb-kinetic, ideomotor, and conceptual) usually encompasses pantomiming real object use and performing object-related and non–object-related gestures to command and after a demonstration.[15,30] Comprehensive praxis assessment addresses various sites (face and upper and lower limbs), possible limb asymmetry, action type (communicative, object-related), various conditions (to verbal command, to imitation) and error types (spatial, sequential).[31] Because most apraxia tests do not encompass all apraxia

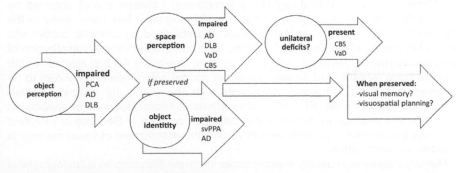

Fig. 3. Visuospatial function assessment.

subtypes,[31] they have limited value in the differential diagnosis of YOD. Praxis evaluation in YOD individuals should be mandatory, as unilateral limb-kinetic/ideomotor apraxia is a core feature of CBS. It may be accompanied by alien limb phenomenon, intermanual conflict, and mirror movements. Also, ideomotor apraxia may be an early sign of young-onset AD (YOAD), particularly of PCA and the apraxic variant. Additionally, conceptual apraxia (loss of gesture meaning) occurs in svPPA (**Table 3**).

According to Hodges,[15] dressing, constructional (both spatially based), and speech apraxias (affecting only speech-related oral movements) cannot be considered classic apraxias mentioned above. Nevertheless, these disorders may also appear in YOD. Dressing apraxia, which is a part of most instrumental activities of daily living inventories,[13] is evaluated mainly based on the caregiver's interview. Of note, although this type of apraxia is typical for the early stages of PCA and CBS, it may also appear in late stages of all dementias.

Assessment of constructional apraxia (see section on visuospatial assessment) is based mainly on drawing (copying and spontaneous) or block assembling tasks, and its impairment predominates in YOAD (especially PCA) and CBS. By comparison, apraxia of speech is a core symptom of nfvPPA[20,21] but may also occur in CBS. It should be evaluated along with language assessment (see section on language assessment).

MEMORY ASSESSMENT

Most patients complain about poor memory.[15] However, although some memory problems in YOD may indeed be amnesic in nature, most patients typically present with nonmemory deficits, even patients with YOAD in whom executive dysfunction often predominates.[32] In fact, a pure amnesic syndrome in YOD is likely to occur mostly in the context of substance-related dementia[33] or in paraneoplastic or infectious disorders (which are not considered in this report). In many individuals with YOD, defective performance on memory tests is secondary to other deficits, such as attention/working memory problems (eg, in DLB or HD), language (eg, in PPA syndromes), or executive function (eg, in frontotemporal dementia [FTD] or PSP).

Despite lack of predominant episodic memory problems in most YOD syndromes, the assessment of these problems significantly adds to the differential diagnosis of YOD. Specifically, the profile of episodic memory test performance may indicate the underlying cognitive mechanism(s) of poor memory performance (eg, amnestic/encoding vs executive/retrieval), often characteristic of a particular type of YOD.[34] For example, because the provision of a cue (helping encoding and retrieval processes) significantly improves the memory scores of patients with lesions affecting the frontal and fronto-striatal regions, a comparison between scores obtained on delayed free recall and on delayed cued recall/recognition has been useful in the differential diagnosis between AD (typically characterized by amnesic profile) and non-AD dementias (see **Table 2**).[1] Further, temporal gradient (better recollection of remote than recent memories), which is typical for late-onset AD and alcohol-related brain damage (ARBD), and to some extent in normal aging, has been shown to be reversed in svPPA. Moreover, in patients with the pathology affecting frontal-subcortical circuitries (eg, FTD, HD) poor retrieval of information may be associated with defective strategy formation and impaired chronology.[13] Because of profound language impairment in patients with PPA, only the assessment of visual memory is feasible and informative.

Memory assessment usually encompasses interview (focusing on autobiographical memory and recollection of current news), observation (retention of instructions during

Table 3
Praxis profile in selected YOD syndromes in contrast to late onset Alzheimer's disease

Type of YOD	Fantomiming Object Use	Performing Symbolic Gestures to Command	Recognizing the Meaning of Gestures	Imitating Examiner's Hand Postures	Performing Sequential Movements	Cause of Impairment
CBS	Impaired	Impaired	Preserved	Severe unilateral impairment (mostly pronounced in finger postures)	Impaired	Generalized gesture output processing[a]
PCA	Initially preserved	Preserved	Impaired	Impaired	Impaired	Visual gesture analysis[a]
svPPA/Semantic dementia	Depends on object knowledge	Impaired	Impaired	Spared	Spared	Action semantics (conceptual)[a]
bvFTD & PSP	Spared or concrete errors	Spared or concrete errors	Spared	Spared	Impaired	Sequential organization of action
DLB & Late-onset Alzheimer's disease	Impaired	Relatively preserved	Relatively preserved	Impaired (especially in terms of positioning hand in relation to the body)	Impaired	Visual gesture analysis & (to a lesser extent) action semantics[a]

The "Command" header spans the columns: Performing Symbolic Gestures to Command, Recognizing the Meaning of Gestures, Imitating Examiner's Hand Postures.

[a] Typology from Bickerton et al,[10] 2012.

testing), and performance on formal memory tests. Early verbal episodic memory impairment is best detected with the use of word list learning (at least 10 words and 3 learning trails), with delayed free recall and cued recall or recognition.[1] The analysis of the learning curve is particularly useful in the differential diagnosis, for example, plateau curve is observed in patients with frontal lobe dysfunctions who also tend to randomly recall words from the list.

Working memory—the ability to actively hold and manipulate the information in mind—is vulnerable to dysfunction in most YOD syndromes. Poor immediate verbal recall is particularly deficient in lvPPA,[20,21] whereas immediate visual recall is severely compromised in PCA[26] and DLB.

In general, most patients have predominant problems with verbal memory, whereas visual memory is typically severely disturbed only in individuals with conditions affecting more posterior brain regions, especially when right temporal-parietal-occipital areas are involved.

Semantic memory assessment (famous faces recognition, word comprehension, and associative verbal and visual tasks), also a part of language testing (naming and verbal fluency), is strongly recommended in the differential diagnosis of YOD, particularly frontotemporal lobar degeneration. To determine if a poor performance on naming or verbal fluency tasks is driven by a more general semantic impairment, as in svPPA, visual semantics needs to be assessed with the use of an association task from Sydney Language Battery.[35] Except for the svPPA and later stages of AD (anterior temporal lobe involvement), semantic memory is spared during the early stages of other types of YOD, although it often declines with the disease duration.

Deficits in procedural learning are typical for YOD with subcortical involvement, especially for PD,[36] and concern the acquisition of both motor (eg, rotor-pursuit task) and cognitive (eg, mirror reading) procedures. However, in the clinical context usually only motor programming with Luria fist-edge-palm is administered.

Selective testing of verbal encoding/recall (especially without recognition trial), although useful in screening for memory problems in the elderly population, is of little use in the differential diagnosis of YOD, unless the testing is integrated into a full cognitive profile.

EXECUTIVE FUNCTION ASSESSMENT

Executive function assessment is the most complex part of neuropsychological examination, and executive deficits are common in YOD (**Fig. 4**). Initiation difficulties, manifesting as prolonged latency to provide answers, difficulty at the beginning of each new task (especially with striking improvement afterward, even on harder items), and poor verbal fluency in the context of good confrontation naming are suggestive of subcortical or fronto-striatal involvement.[37] Poor initiation usually coexists with apathy and depression.[38] Thus, integration of neuropsychological and neuropsychiatric data is crucial.

Difficulties in planning, frequently seen as a consequence of frontal dysfunction, may be formally assessed with tower tasks, although for many individuals such tasks are too challenging. Impaired planning can also be observed during clock drawing (with the executive clock drawing task, it is possible to discriminate between poor planning and poor construction caused by perceptual failure)[39] or copying of the complex figure[19] (ie, impaired copy in the context of good performance on spatial tasks not requiring planning, such as spatial subtests from VOSP). Sequential reasoning may be assessed through picture arrangement task that is not timed or perceptually complex.[40]

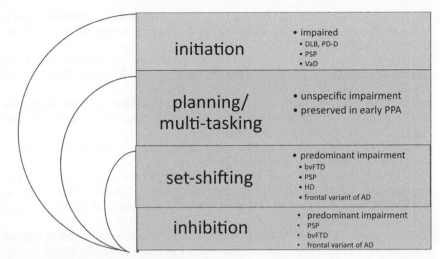

Fig. 4. Executive function assessment.

Mental set shifting is best assessed with low-demanding stimuli, such as Weigl block sorting[41] or The Brixton Spatial Anticipation Test,[42] as failures on complex tasks such as card sorting tests are difficult to interpret because of multiple cognitive demands (especially working and episodic memory). Marked cognitive rigidity may manifest throughout the testing as persistent verbal and motor perseverations.[19]

A patient impulsively providing the first answer that comes to mind is often a sign of severely defective inhibition, particularly when this is done repeatedly. On testing, it may be quantified with go/no-go and conflicting tasks. Mild inhibition problems may emerge only in high-demanding tasks such as the Stroop Interference test.[43] Patients who present with both poor inhibition and marked perseveration may also fail to produce simple alternate designs, as they may perseverate details in tasks such as copying a complex figure. A positive clapping sign; any instances of echolalia, imitation, or utilization behavior; or any other environmental dependency behaviors are highly suggestive of frontal[44] or fronto-parietal dysfunction.[45]

SUMMARY

YOD is an umbrella term encompassing a wide range of disorders, but most of them fall within FTD or YOAD spectrum. Thus, the neuropsychological profile of YOD is very heterogeneous. Apart from ARBD, a true amnestic syndrome is unusual for YOD. Language, executive, visual, or praxis deficits are frequently the presenting features of a YOD, and these impairments can be brought into full view by neuropsychological tests. Whenever YOD is suspected, fairly comprehensive neuropsychological testing is mandatory for diagnosis and further management.

REFERENCES

1. Sorbi S, Hort J, Erkinjuntti T, et al. EFNS-ENS Guidelines on the diagnosis and management of disorders associated with dementia. Eur J Neurol 2012;19: 1159–79.
2. Jacova C, Kertesz A, Blair M, et al. Neuropsychological testing and assessment for dementia. Alzheimers Dement 2007;3:299–317.

3. Snowden JS, Thompson JC, Stopford CL, et al. The clinical diagnosis of early-onset dementias: diagnostic accuracy and clinicopathological relationships. Brain 2011;134:2478–92.

4. Folstein MF, Folstein SE, McHugh PR. "Mini-mental state". A practical method for grading the cognitive state of patients for the clinician. J Psychiatr Res 1975;12: 189–98.

5. Hsieh S, Schubert S, Hoon C, et al. Validation of the Addenbrooke's Cognitive Examination III in frontotemporal dementia and Alzheimer's disease. Dement Geriatr Cogn Disord 2013;36:242–50.

6. Jurica PJ, Leitten CL, Mattis S. Dementia rating scale—2 professional manual. Lutz (FL): Psychological Assessment Resources; 2001.

7. Abrahams S, Newton J, Niven E, et al. Screening for cognition and behaviour changes in ALS. Amyotroph Lateral Scler Frontotemporal Degener 2014;15:9–14.

8. Cullen B, O'Neill B, Evans JJ, et al. A review of screening tests for cognitive impairment. J Neurol Neurosurg Psychiatry 2007;78:790–9.

9. Bak TH, Rogers TT, Crawford LM, et al. Cognitive bedside assessment in atypical parkinsonian syndromes. J Neurol Neurosurg Psychiatry 2005;76:420–2.

10. Bickerton WL, Riddoch MJ, Samson D, et al. Systematic assessment of apraxia and functional predictions from the Birmingham Cognitive Screen. J Neurol Neurosurg Psychiatry 2012;83:513–21.

11. Dubois B, Slachevsky A, Litvan I, et al. The FAB: a frontal assessment battery at bedside. Neurology 2000;55:1621–6.

12. Torralva T, Roca M, Gleichgerrcht E, et al. INECO Frontal Screening (IFS): a brief, sensitive, and specific tool to assess executive functions in dementia. J Int Neuropsychol Soc 2009;15:777–86.

13. Lezak MD, Howieson DB, Bigler ED, et al. Neuropsychological assessment. 5th edition. New York: Oxford University Press; 2012.

14. Kertesz A, Nadkarni N, Davidson W, et al. The frontal behavioral inventory in the differential diagnosis of frontotemporal dementia. J Int Neuropsychol Soc 2000;6:460–8.

15. Hodges JR. Cognitive assessment for clinicians. 2nd edition. New York: Oxford University Press; 2007.

16. Rascovsky K, Hodges JR, Knopman D, et al. Sensitivity of revised diagnostic criteria for the behavioural variant of frontotemporal dementia. Brain 2011;134: 2456–77.

17. Ford AH. Neuropsychiatric aspects of dementia. Maturitas 2014;79:209–15.

18. Doubleday EK, Snowden JS, Varma AR, et al. Qualitative performance characteristics differentiate dementia with Lewy bodies and Alzheimer's disease. J Neurol Neurosurg Psychiatry 2002;72:602–7.

19. Thompson JC, Stopford CL, Snowden JS, et al. Qualitative neuropsychological performance characteristics in frontotemporal dementia and Alzheimer's disease. J Neurol Neurosurg Psychiatry 2005;76:920–7.

20. Gorno-Tempini ML, Hillis AE, Weintraub S, et al. Classification of primary progressive aphasia and its variants. Neurology 2011;76:1006–14.

21. Harciarek M, Kertesz A. Primary progressive aphasias and their contribution to the contemporary knowledge about the brain-language relationship. Neuropsychol Rev 2011;21:271–87.

22. Josephs KA, Duffy JR. Apraxia of speech and nonfluent aphasia: a new clinical marker for corticobasal degeneration and progressive supranuclear palsy. Curr Opin Neurol 2008;21:688–92.

23. Neary D, Snowden JS, Gustafson L, et al. Frontotemporal lobar degeneration: a consensus on clinical diagnostic criteria. Neurology 1998;51:1546–54.

24. Rosser A, Hodges JR. Initial letter and semantic category fluency in Alzheimer's disease, Huntington's disease, and progressive supranuclear palsy. J Neurol Neurosurg Psychiatry 1994;57:1389–94.
25. Warrington EK, Merle J. Visual object and space perception test battery. United Kingdom: Thames Valley Company; 1991.
26. Aresi A, Giovagnoli AR. The role of neuropsychology in distinguishing the posterior cortical atrophy syndrome and Alzheimer's disease. J Alzheimers Dis 2009; 18:65–70.
27. Josephs KA, Whitwell JL, Knopman DS, et al. Two distinct subtypes of right temporal variant frontotemporal dementia. Neurology 2009;73:1443–50.
28. Boyd CD, Tierney M, Wassermann EM, et al. Visuoperception test predicts pathologic diagnosis of Alzheimer disease in corticobasal syndrome. Neurology 2014;83:510–9.
29. Mathew R, Bak TH, Hodges JR. Diagnostic criteria for corticobasal syndrome: a comparative study. J Neurol Neurosurg Psychiatr 2012;83:405–10.
30. Heilman KM. Apraxia. Continuum (Minneap Minn) 2010;16:86–98.
31. Dovern A, Fink GR, Weiss PH. Diagnosis and treatment of upper limb apraxia. J Neurol 2012;259:1269–83.
32. Koedam EL, Lauffer V, van der Vlies AE, et al. Early-versus late-onset Alzheimer's disease: more than age alone. J Alzheimers Dis 2010;19:1401–8.
33. Oslin D, Atkinson RM, Smith DM, et al. Alcohol related dementia: proposed clinical criteria. Int J Geriatr Psychiatry 1998;13:203–12.
34. Pasquier F. Early diagnosis of dementia: neuropsychology. J Neurol 1999;246: 6–15.
35. Savage S, Hsieh S, Leslie F, et al. Distinguishing subtypes in primary progressive aphasia: application of the Sydney language battery. Dement Geriatr Cogn Disord 2013;35:208–18.
36. Foerde K, Shohamy D. The role of the basal ganglia in learning and memory: insight from Parkinson's disease. Neurobiol Learn Mem 2011;96:624–36.
37. Duke LM, Kaszniak AW. Executive control functions in degenerative dementias: a comparative review. Neuropsychol Rev 2000;10:75–99.
38. Grossi D, Santangelo G, Barbarulo AM, et al. Apathy and related executive syndromes in dementia associated with Parkinson's disease and in Alzheimer's disease. Behav Neurol 2013;27:515–22.
39. Royall DR, Cordes JA, Polk M. CLOX: an executive clock drawing task. J Neurol Neurosurg Psychiatr 1998;64:588–94.
40. Snowden J, Craufurd D, Griffiths H, et al. Longitudinal evaluation of cognitive disorder in Huntington's disease. J Int Neuropsychol Soc 2001;7:33–44.
41. Weigl E. On the psychology of so-called processes of abstraction. J Norm Soc Psych 1941;36:3–33.
42. Burgess PW, Shallice T. Bizarre responses, rule detection and frontal lobe lesions. Cortex 1996;32:241–59.
43. Stroop JR. Studies of interference in serial verbal reactions. J Exp Psychol 1935; 18:643–62.
44. Ghosh A, Dutt A, Bhargava P, et al. Environmental dependency behaviours in frontotemporal dementia: have we been underrating them? J Neurol 2013;260: 861–8.
45. Lagarde J, Valabregue R, Corvol JC, et al. The clinical and anatomical heterogeneity of environmental dependency phenomena. J Neurol 2013;260:2262–70.

Brain Imaging in the Differential Diagnosis of Young-Onset Dementias

HyungSub Shim, MD[a],*, Maria J. Ly, BA[b], Sarah K. Tighe, MD[b]

KEYWORDS

- Young-onset dementia • Alzheimer disease • Frontotemporal dementia • MRI • PET
- Parkinson-plus disorders

KEY POINTS

- No single neuroimaging modality is diagnostic of young-onset dementia (YOD), but specific imaging patterns are suggestive of certain causes.
- MRI is routinely recommended in the workup of YOD.
- Functional nuclear imaging provides in vivo measures of brain functioning and can shed light on the presence of certain neurodegenerative processes.
- Structural and functional neuroimaging are important in the workup for YOD and can inform important aspects of dementia care such as the underlying disease, treatment, and prognosis.

INTRODUCTION

Young-onset dementia (YOD) is defined as dementia with onset of symptoms before 65 years of age. YOD has key epidemiologic differences from late-onset dementia, primarily in that Alzheimer disease (AD) accounts for a much smaller percentage of cases. Additionally, many genetic forms of dementia manifest as YOD.[1] Despite being far less prevalent than late-onset dementia,[2,3] YOD causes a disproportionate burden on society, families, and individuals owing to a variety of factors, such as the considerable loss of productivity for both patients and caregivers.[4,5]

Relatively predictable links between specific syndromes and pathologies have been determined, although the correspondence is far from perfect.[6–8] For instance, in a study of 40 subjects with the clinical diagnosis of corticobasal syndrome (CBS), only 14% had the corresponding corticobasal degeneration pathology on autopsy.[9]

Disclosures: None.
a Department of Neurology, University of Iowa Hospitals and Clinics, University of Iowa Carver College of Medicine, 200 Hawkins Drive, Iowa City, IA 52242, USA; b Department of Psychiatry, University of Iowa Carver College of Medicine, 200 Hawkins Drive, Iowa City, IA 52242, USA
* Corresponding author.
E-mail address: hyungsubshim@gmail.com

Psychiatr Clin N Am 38 (2015) 281–294
http://dx.doi.org/10.1016/j.psc.2015.01.007
0193-953X/15/$ – see front matter © 2015 Elsevier Inc. All rights reserved.

Abbreviations	
AD	Alzheimer disease
bvFTD	Behavioral variant frontotemporal dementia
CBS	Corticobasal syndrome
CJD	Creutzfeldt-Jakob disease
DAT	Dopamine transporter
DLB	Dementia with Lewy bodies
FDG	[^{18}F]-2-fluoro-2-deoxy-D-glucose
FTLD	Frontotemporal lobar degeneration
LOAD	Late-onset Alzheimer disease
LPA	Logopenic progressive aphasia
PCA	Posterior cortical atrophy
PIB	Pittsburgh compound B
PNFA	Progressive nonfluent aphasia
PPA	Primary progressive aphasia
PSP	Progressive supranuclear palsy
SD	Semantic dementia
SPECT	Single-photon emission computed tomography
VaD	Vascular dementia
YOAD	Young-onset Alzheimer disease
YOD	Young-onset dementia

Of the studies exploring these links, those that used relatively fine-grain neuropsychological test results and imaging findings had the highest sensitivities and specificities.[6] This speaks to the importance of neuroimaging and other testing modalities for helping to enrich and support the clinical diagnosis.

This article reviews the role of neuroimaging in the differential diagnosis of YOD. This is intended to be a high-yield article to guide clinicians in the utility and diagnostic evaluation of YOD. The focus is on clinical, rather than pathologic, diagnoses of YOD. However, it also addresses how imaging might help predict an underlying pathologic condition.

DIAGNOSTIC APPROACH

The differential diagnosis of YOD is quite broad, so a systematic approach to the workup is recommended. After a careful clinical assessment, structural imaging is necessary for 2 reasons: (1) to rule out structural lesions (eg, tumors or hydrocephalus) that may cause cognitive decline and (2) to inform the differential diagnosis. The American Academy of Neurology recommends structural neuroimaging at least once for all patients with dementia.[10] This article focuses on MRI. Other imaging modalities include functional nuclear imaging, specifically PET and single-photon emission computed tomography (SPECT). Common PET tracers are [^{18}F]-2-fluoro-2-deoxy-D-glucose (FDG), a marker of cerebral glucose metabolism, as well as Pittsburgh compound B (PIB) and ^{18}F-florbetapir, both markers of β-amyloid. Characteristic neuroimaging patterns are helpful in the diagnostic workup of YOD (see later discussion) (Table 1).

ALZHEIMER DISEASE

AD represents the most prevalent cause of YOD. Of the 5.4 million Americans affected by AD, approximately 4% to 5% experience onset before age 65.[11] Unlike late-onset AD (LOAD), which presents with prominent memory loss, young-onset AD (YOAD) has a relative sparing of memory in early stages, whereas cognitive

Table 1
Young-onset dementia diagnoses and their characteristic imaging findings

Diagnosis	MRI Findings	Functional Nuclear Imaging Findings
AD	Mesial temporal atrophy, posterior > anterior atrophy, thalamic and striatal atrophy	FDG-PET: widespread cortical hypometabolism especially in temporal and parietal cortices, deep gray structures
Behavioral variant frontotemporal dementia	Anterior predominant atrophy, may be asymmetric	FDG-PET: frontotemporal hypometabolism, especially early in disease, even in absence of atrophy
Dementia with Lewy bodies	No cortical atrophy, mild midbrain atrophy	FDG-PET: posterior temporoparietal and occipital hypometabolism. dopamine transporter–SPECT: decreased dopamine transport in striatum
Posterior cortical atrophy syndrome	Posterior occipitoparietal and inferior-posterior temporal atrophy, right > left	FDG-PET right occipitoparietal and occipitotemporal hypometabolism
Primary progressive aphasia	Left > right atrophy	FDG-PET pattern similar to MRI in all subtypes
Progressive nonfluent aphasia	Left frontal atrophy, may extend to include temporal or parietal areas	Amyloid-PET usually negative
Semantic dementia	Left > right anterior temporal atrophy	Amyloid-PET usually negative
Logopenic progressive aphasia	Diffuse left cortical atrophy, maximal in temporoparietal junction	Amyloid-PET usually positive
Progressive supranuclear palsy	Severe midbrain atrophy (hummingbird and morning glory signs)	FDG-PET shows brainstem hypometabolism
CBS	Asymmetric frontal atrophy ± more widespread atrophy	FDG-PET asymmetric hypometabolism in basal ganglia and parietal cortex

dysfunction rapidly progresses in domains such as visuospatial functioning, praxis, executive functioning, and attentional processing.[12] Nearly 20% of YOAD are caused by autosomal-dominant mutations in presenilin 1, presenilin 2, or amyloid precursor protein genes.[11]

In addition to the classic pattern of symmetric atrophy predominantly in the mesial temporal lobes, more widespread atrophy is often seen earlier in YOAD compared with LOAD. Neocortical atrophy in YOAD occurs in the association cortices[13] and, more specifically, in the temporoparietal junction.[14] Thalamic and striatal volume loss has also been noted in YOAD.[15] Visually determined mesial temporal atrophy (**Fig. 1**), as well as a pattern of cortical atrophy that is greater in the posterior parietal lobes than in the frontal lobes, have high sensitivity and specificity in differentiating AD from controls and frontotemporal lobar degeneration (FTLD).[16] More specific patterns of neocortical atrophy are also well-described[17] but generally present differently clinically (see later discussion).

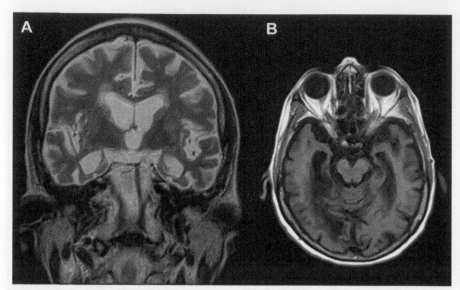

Fig. 1. MRI of a patient with AD. Coronal T2 (*A*) and axial T1 (*B*) images, both showing severe bilateral mesial temporal atrophy.

LOAD is characterized by reduced glucose metabolism in the parietotemporal, frontal, and posterior cingulate cortices (**Fig. 2**). In comparison to LOAD, the FDG-PET profile of YOAD is characterized by more severe hypometabolism of these structures, as well as involvement of the basal ganglia and thalamus.[18,19] Based on studies of PIB-PET uptake, global measures of β-amyloid tend to be similar in YOAD and LOAD; however, YOAD may show uptake in the basal ganglia and thalamus.[20] PET has a role in discriminating AD from other YOD causes (see later discussion).

VASCULAR DEMENTIA

Vascular dementia (VaD) is defined as cognitive decline following one or more cardiovascular events, such as stroke. VaD is a leading cause of dementia overall but less so in YOD.[3] Nevertheless, familial causes may occur earlier in life. With usual onset age in the 30s, cerebral autosomal dominant arteriopathy with subcortical infarcts and leukoencephalopathy is one such example.[21]

Given the heterogeneity of its underlying pathologic condition, VaD lacks hallmark structural or functional neuroimaging findings. MRI evidence of severe and/or pervasive cerebrovascular disease supports the diagnosis. The most common pattern is widespread small vessel ischemic disease (**Fig. 3**) but single or multiple infarcts or hemorrhages may also be seen.

BEHAVIORAL VARIANT FRONTOTEMPORAL DEMENTIA

FTLD is the second-most common cause of YOD, affecting approximately 15 to 22 per 100,000 individuals.[22–24] Multiple clinical syndromes are caused by the FTLD family of diseases. Behavioral variant frontotemporal dementia (bvFTD) is the most common and is marked by progressive personality changes and executive dysfunction.[25]

BvFTD has been associated with a variety of patterns of atrophy, including its absence.[26] These include relatively isolated (and often severe) atrophy of the frontal lobes; atrophy of both the frontal and temporal lobes; and more widespread atrophy

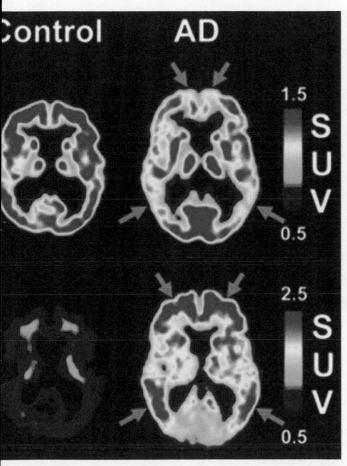

and FDG-PET scans from control and AD participants. Arrows indicate metabolism (FDG) or typical amyloid deposition on PIB-PET. (*From* Co-rly detection of Alzheimer's disease using PiB and FDG PET. Neurobiol ; with permission.)

ral, and parietal cortices, as well as deep gray nuclei **(Fig. 4)**.[27,28] ns of atrophy may predict the underlying pathology.[7,8] In general, anterior, predominance of atrophy should raise suspicion for AD. erable variability in structural findings, PET plays an important role vFTD. Early in the disease, symmetric frontal hypometabolism can absence of visible atrophy.[29,30] Later in the disease course, the ces spread to the parietal and temporal cortices.[29,31]

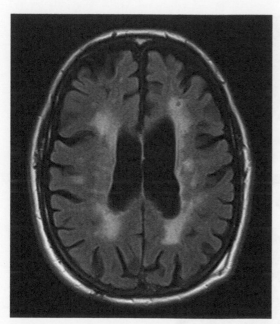

of a patient with VaD. Fluid attenuation inversion recovery (FLAIR) imaging
spread white matter small vessel ischemic disease.

clinically diagnosed with PCA historically had, as the name suggests, atro-
terior cortical areas (**Fig. 5**). The visual association cortices in the occipital,
d inferior and posterior temporal lobes seem to be most affected, with a
ance of atrophy on the right compared with typical AD cases. Conversely,
pocampus is relatively spared compared with typical AD.[33] A similar asym-
en on FDG-PET in PCA. Reduced metabolism in the right occipitoparietal
inguishes PCA from AD,[34] whereas hypometabolism in the right lateral

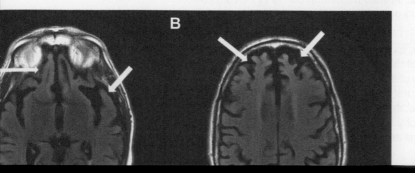

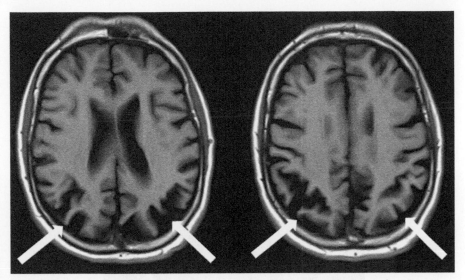

Fig. 5. MRI of a patient with PCA syndrome. T1 axial image with arrows showing severe bilateral posterior parietal atrophy with a slight right predominance.

temporooccipital cortex differentiates PCA from DLB.[35] Over time, the specificity of these findings tends to fade as the underlying disease progresses such that the imaging profile resembles that of typical AD[36] or CBS.[37]

PRIMARY PROGRESSIVE APHASIA

The hallmark of primary progressive aphasia (PPA) is the insidious onset of progressive language impairment with relative preservation of memory and other cognitive domains.[38] Usually PPA begins before the age of 65.[39] PPA has been classified into 3 variants: progressive nonfluent aphasia (PNFA), logopenic progressive aphasia (LPA), and semantic dementia (SD).[40] Whereas SD is predictably caused by FTLD pathology, PNFA and LPA have variable underlying pathology, with FTLD and AD being the most common, respectively.[39,41]

Each subtype of PPA has its own signature pattern of atrophy. SD has the most easily identified and consistent pattern, with left greater than right anterior temporal atrophy (**Fig. 6**). In LPA, atrophy is seen diffusely throughout the left hemisphere, maximal in the temporoparietal junction. In PNFA, atrophy is seen in left frontal regions, including the inferior frontal gyrus and the dorsolateral prefrontal cortex. Some temporoparietal or right-sided atrophy may also be seen.[42,43] FDG-PET findings in PPA typically mirror these volumetric changes.[44]

Combining clinical subtyping with structural MRI may be helpful in determining the underlying pathology in the nonfluent subtypes of PPA. In general, involvement of the posterior superior temporal lobe is predictive of AD, whereas atrophy in other perisylvian regions, the dorsolateral prefrontal cortex, and insula are predictive of non-AD pathology.[43] Of the subtypes, LPA most commonly has positive amyloid reactivity.[44,45]

DEMENTIA WITH LEWY BODIES

Although DLB is a common cause of dementia overall, it only accounts for approximately 0.4% to 2% of cases of YOD.[3] Most cases of DLB are sporadic, though genetic

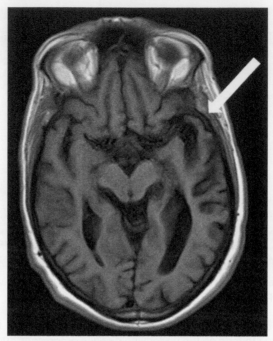

Fig. 6. MRI of a patient with SD, a subtype of PPA. T1 axial image with arrow showing severe left greater than right anterior temporal atrophy.

cases have been reported.[46,47] Core symptoms of DLB include sudden fluctuations in cognition and attention, visual hallucinations, and parkinsonism.

No clear pattern of cortical atrophy has been reported in DLB.[48] Analysis of the brainstem shows volume loss compared with AD, specifically in the dorsal midbrain.[49,50] Posterior parietotemporal and occipital hypometabolism on FDG-PET is characteristic of DLB,[48,51] with occipital hypometabolism discriminating DLB from AD with 90% sensitivity and 80% specificity.[51] Given the hallmark nigrostriatal dopaminergic degeneration of parkinsonian syndromes, dopamine transporter (DAT)-SPECT has received considerable attention in DLB. Abnormal DAT-SPECT scans have a sensitivity and specificity in the diagnosis of DLB of approximately 75% and 90%, respectively.[52]

PROGRESSIVE SUPRANUCLEAR PALSY

Progressive supranuclear palsy (PSP) is the second-most common neurodegenerative syndrome causing parkinsonism, affecting approximately 6.0 to 6.4 individuals per 100,000. The average age of onset is 63.[53] PSP is manifested by downward gaze palsy, progressive rigidity, parkinsonism with early falls, hypophonia, and executive dysfunction.[54] Nearly all cases of PSP are caused by a pathology involving tauopathy (FTLD-tau).[55]

Classic imaging findings in PSP involve the midbrain. In sagittal views, the midbrain can be seen as markedly diminished in size compared with the pons. This is known as the penguin, or hummingbird, sign due to the resemblance of the thinned midbrain to the head and long, thin beak of a bird. In axial views, midbrain atrophy causes a scooped out appearance (the morning glory sign) with the cerebral peduncles looking wide-spaced in comparison (**Fig. 7**).[55] The presence of hypometabolism in the midbrain on FDG-PET is another indication of PSP and can help differentiate the condition from other parkinsonian syndromes.[56]

CORTICOBASAL SYNDROME

CBS is a rare neurodegenerative disorder characterized by an insidious onset of asymmetric cortical and extrapyramidal dysfunction, with an average symptom onset at 63.7 years.[57] Symptoms of CBS usually include parkinsonism, executive dysfunction, asymmetric apraxia, myoclonic jerking, and dystonia. The underlying pathology of CBS is variable, with major contribution from FTLD-tau, as well as AD.[58]

Typically, patients with CBS have asymmetric parietal atrophy, as well as hypometabolism in the basal ganglia and parietal cortex contralateral to the affected side.[56,59] However, neuroimaging correlates of this syndrome have proven to be more variable, with structural neuroimaging only consistently showing frontal (premotor and supplemental motor) atrophy contralateral to the side of worse rigidity or apraxia.[9,58] In addition, CBS has been defined by increased metabolic activity in the basal ganglia and cortical regions ipsilateral to the affected side.[60,61] If the atrophy includes both temporoparietal regions, AD is more likely, whereas findings in the literature associated with FTLD pathology are less clear.[9,58,62]

OTHER IMAGING FINDINGS

MRI can also be useful to evaluate for other causes of YOD, especially when there is significant family history, subacute onset, or suspicion for multisystem disease. Other structural changes that can be evident on MRI include severe atrophy of the caudate and putamen in Huntington disease,[63] basal ganglionic calcifications from Fahr disease,[64] widespread volume loss in the setting of repeated head injury (chronic traumatic encephalopathy),[65] disproportionately enlarged ventricles from normal pressure

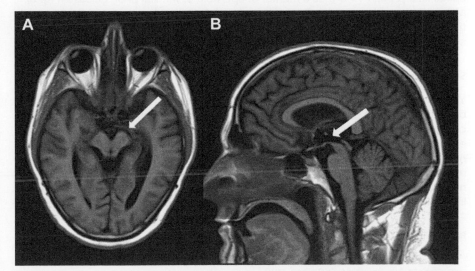

Fig. 7. MRI of a patient with PSP. Axial T1 image (A) with arrow showing scooped out appearance to midbrain, morning glory sign, and sagittal T1 image (B) with arrow showing thinning of midbrain as well, hummingbird sign.

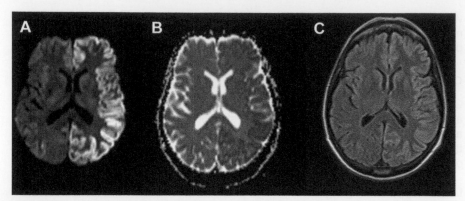

Fig. 8. MRI of a patient with biopsy-proven CJD. Diffusion-weighted imaging (*A*) shows hyperintensities in the striatum, thalamus, and cortex, more striking on the left. Apparent diffusion coefficient map (*B*) shows dark areas corresponding to the diffusion-weighted imaging change, indicating diffusion restriction. The FLAIR image (*C*) also shows hyperintensity but not as intensely.

hydrocephalus,[66] signs of low intracranial pressure (frontotemporal brain sagging syndrome),[67] meningeal and parenchymal granulomatous disease in neurosarcoidosis,[68] demyelinating plaques in multiple sclerosis,[69] or callosal microinfarcts in Susac syndrome.[70] Rarely, inherited metabolic diseases, such as adrenoleukodystrophy and metachromatic leukodystrophy, present in adulthood, usually with widespread white matter involvement.[69]

In the case of rapidly progressive dementias, MRI is supplanting cerebrospinal fluid in the diagnosis of prion disease.[71] The presence of widespread diffusion restriction (visible on diffusion-weighted imaging and apparent diffusion coefficient map images) in the deep and cortical gray matter is now more sensitive and specific than cerebrospinal fluid protein 14-3-3 as a marker of sporadic or familial prion disease (**Fig. 8**).[72] MRI may also help uncover signs of thiamine deficiency,[73] paraneoplastic encephalitis,[74] or sequelae of infections such as human immunodeficiency virus and syphilis.[75,76]

SUMMARY

YOD is a broad category of diseases that affect adults before the age of 65, with devastating effects on individuals, families, and communities. Neuroimaging plays a clear and ever-expanding role in the workup of these diseases. With a careful clinical evaluation in hand, MRI and PET imaging can enrich and support the clinical diagnosis. Given the lack of one-to-one correlation between clinical and pathologic diagnoses, imaging can also help to predict the underlying condition of YOD, which in turn helps determine prognosis and treatment. Continuing advances in neuroimaging will likely play a major role in the understanding of these diseases and their management.

REFERENCES

1. Rossor MN, Fox NC, Mummery CJ, et al. The diagnosis of young-onset dementia. Lancet Neurol 2010;9(8):793–806.
2. Lambert MA, Bickel H, Prince M, et al. Estimating the burden of early onset dementia; systematic review of disease prevalence. Eur J Neurol 2014;21(4):563–9.

3. Vieira RT, Caixeta L, Machado S, et al. Epidemiology of early-onset dementia: a review of the literature. Clin Pract Epidemiol Ment Health 2013;9:88–95.
4. Werner P, Stein-Shvachman I, Korczyn AD. Early onset dementia: clinical and social aspects. Int psychogeriatr 2009;21(4):631–6.
5. van Vliet D, de Vugt ME, Bakker C, et al. Impact of early onset dementia on caregivers: a review. Int J Geriatr Psychiatry 2010;25(11):1091–100.
6. Snowden JS, Thompson JC, Stopford CL, et al. The clinical diagnosis of early-onset dementias: diagnostic accuracy and clinicopathological relationships. Brain 2011;134(Pt 9):2478–92.
7. Rohrer JD, Geser F, Zhou J, et al. TDP-43 subtypes are associated with distinct atrophy patterns in frontotemporal dementia. Neurology 2010;75(24):2204–11.
8. Rohrer JD, Lashley T, Schott JM, et al. Clinical and neuroanatomical signatures of tissue pathology in frontotemporal lobar degeneration. Brain 2011;134(Pt 9):2565–81.
9. Lee SE, Rabinovici GD, Mayo MC, et al. Clinicopathological correlations in corticobasal degeneration. Ann Neurol 2011;70(2):327–40.
10. Knopman DS, DeKosky ST, Cummings JL, et al. Practice parameter: diagnosis of dementia (an evidence-based review). report of the quality standards subcommittee of the American academy of neurology. Neurology 2001;56(9):1143–53.
11. Alzheimer's A. 2014 Alzheimer's disease facts and figures. Alzheimers Demen 2014;10(2):e47–92.
12. Ishii K, Kono A, Sasaki H, et al. Fully automatic diagnostic system for early- and late-onset mild Alzheimer's disease using FDG PET and 3D-SSP. Eur J Nucl Med Mol Imaging 2006;33(5):575–83.
13. Cho H, Jeon S, Kang SJ, et al. Longitudinal changes of cortical thickness in early- versus late-onset Alzheimer's disease. Neurobiol Aging 2013;34(7):1921.e9–15.
14. Frisoni GB, Testa C, Sabattoli F, et al. Structural correlates of early and late onset Alzheimer's disease: voxel based morphometric study. J Neurol Neurosurg Psychiatry 2005;76(1):112–4.
15. Cho H, Seo SW, Kim JH, et al. Changes in subcortical structures in early- versus late-onset Alzheimer's disease. Neurobiol Aging 2013;34(7):1740–7.
16. Likeman M, Anderson VM, Stevens JM, et al. Visual assessment of atrophy on magnetic resonance imaging in the diagnosis of pathologically confirmed young-onset dementias. Arch Neurol 2005;62(9):1410–5.
17. Migliaccio R, Agosta F, Rascovsky K, et al. Clinical syndromes associated with posterior atrophy: early age at onset AD spectrum. Neurology 2009;73(19):1571–8.
18. Sakamoto S, Ishii K, Sasaki M, et al. Differences in cerebral metabolic impairment between early and late onset types of Alzheimer's disease. J Neurol Sci 2002;200(1–2):27–32.
19. Kim EJ, Cho SS, Jeong Y, et al. Glucose metabolism in early onset versus late onset Alzheimer's disease: an SPM analysis of 120 patients. Brain 2005;128(Pt 8):1790–801.
20. Cho H, Seo SW, Kim JH, et al. Amyloid deposition in early onset versus late onset Alzheimer's disease. J Alzheimers Dis 2013;35(4):813–21.
21. Choudhary S, McLeod M, Torchia D, et al. Cerebral autosomal dominant arteriopathy with subcortical infarcts and leukoencephalopathy (CADASIL). J Clin Aesthet Dermatol 2013;6(3):29–33.
22. Ratnavalli E, Brayne C, Dawson K, et al. The prevalence of frontotemporal dementia. Neurology 2002;58(11):1615–21.

23. Harvey RJ, Skelton-Robinson M, Rossor MN. The prevalence and causes of dementia in people under the age of 65 years. J Neurol Neurosurg Psychiatry 2003; 74(9):1206–9.

24. Borroni B, Alberici A, Grassi M, et al. Is frontotemporal lobar degeneration a rare disorder? Evidence from a preliminary study in Brescia county, Italy. J Alzheimers Dis 2010;19(1):111–6.

25. Seelaar H, Rohrer JD, Pijnenburg YA, et al. Clinical, genetic and pathological heterogeneity of frontotemporal dementia: a review. J Neurol Neurosurg Psychiatry 2011;82(5):476–86.

26. Koedam EL, Van der Flier WM, Barkhof F, et al. Clinical characteristics of patients with frontotemporal dementia with and without lobar atrophy on MRI. Alzheimer Dis Assoc Disord 2010;24(3):242–7.

27. Diehl-Schmid J, Onur OA, Kuhn J, et al. Imaging frontotemporal lobar degeneration. Curr Neurol Neurosci Rep 2014;14(10):489.

28. Moller C, Dieleman N, van der Flier WM, et al. More atrophy of deep gray matter structures in frontotemporal dementia compared to Alzheimer's disease. J Alzheimers Dis 2015;44:635–47.

29. Diehl-Schmid J, Grimmer T, Drzezga A, et al. Decline of cerebral glucose metabolism in frontotemporal dementia: a longitudinal 18F-FDG-PET-study. Neurobiol Aging 2007;28(1):42–50.

30. Diehl J, Grimmer T, Drzezga A, et al. Cerebral metabolic patterns at early stages of frontotemporal dementia and semantic dementia. A PET study. Neurobiol Aging 2004;25(8):1051–6.

31. Ishii K, Sakamoto S, Sasaki M, et al. Cerebral glucose metabolism in patients with frontotemporal dementia. J Nucl Med 1998;39(11):1875–8.

32. Beh SC, Muthusamy B, Calabresi P, et al. Hiding in plain sight: a closer look at posterior cortical atrophy. Pract Neurol 2015;15:5–13.

33. Lehmann M, Crutch SJ, Ridgway GR, et al. Cortical thickness and voxel-based morphometry in posterior cortical atrophy and typical Alzheimer's disease. Neurobiol Aging 2011;32(8):1466–76.

34. Nestor PJ, Caine D, Fryer TD, et al. The topography of metabolic deficits in posterior cortical atrophy (the visual variant of Alzheimer's disease) with FDG-PET. J Neurol Neurosurg Psychiatry 2003;74(11):1521–9.

35. Spehl TS, Hellwig S, Amtage F, et al. Syndrome-specific patterns of regional cerebral glucose metabolism in posterior cortical atrophy in comparison to dementia with lewy bodies and alzheimer's disease-A [F-18]-Fdg pet study. J Neuroimaging 2014. [Epub ahead of print].

36. Lehmann M, Barnes J, Ridgway GR, et al. Global gray matter changes in posterior cortical atrophy: a serial imaging study. Alzheimers Demen 2012;8(6):502–12.

37. Giorelli M, Losignore NA, Bagnoli J, et al. The progression of posterior cortical atrophy to corticobasal syndrome: lumping or splitting neurodegenerative diseases? Tremor Other Hyperkinet Mov (N Y) 2014;4:244.

38. Mesulam MM. Primary progressive aphasia—a language-based dementia. N Engl J Med 2003;349(16):1535–42.

39. Mesulam MM, Weintraub S, Rogalski EJ, et al. Asymmetry and heterogeneity of Alzheimer's and frontotemporal pathology in primary progressive aphasia. Brain 2014;137(Pt 4):1176–92.

40. Gorno-Tempini ML, Hillis AE, Weintraub S, et al. Classification of primary progressive aphasia and its variants. Neurology 2011;76(11):1006–14.

41. Harris JM, Gall C, Thompson JC, et al. Classification and pathology of primary progressive aphasia. Neurology 2013;81(21):1832–9.

42. Rogalski E, Cobia D, Harrison TM, et al. Progression of language decline and cortical atrophy in subtypes of primary progressive aphasia. Neurology 2011; 76(21):1804–10.
43. Hu WT, McMillan C, Libon D, et al. Multimodal predictors for Alzheimer disease in nonfluent primary progressive aphasia. Neurology 2010;75(7):595–602.
44. Rabinovici GD, Jagust WJ, Furst AJ, et al. Abeta amyloid and glucose metabolism in three variants of primary progressive aphasia. Ann Neurol 2008;64(4): 388–401.
45. Leyton CE, Villemagne VL, Savage S, et al. Subtypes of progressive aphasia: application of the international consensus criteria and validation using beta-amyloid imaging. Brain 2011;134(Pt 10):3030–43.
46. Galvin JE, Lee SL, Perry A, et al. Familial dementia with Lewy bodies: clinicopathologic analysis of two kindreds. Neurology 2002;59(7):1079–82.
47. Tsuang DW, Dalan AM, Eugenio CJ, et al. Familial dementia with lewy bodies: a clinical and neuropathological study of 2 families. Arch Neurol 2002;59(10): 1622–30.
48. Kantarci K, Lowe VJ, Boeve BF, et al. Multimodality imaging characteristics of dementia with Lewy bodies. Neurobiol Aging 2012;33(9):2091–105.
49. Kantarci K, Ferman TJ, Boeve BF, et al. Focal atrophy on MRI and neuropathologic classification of dementia with Lewy bodies. Neurology 2012;79(6): 553–60.
50. Nakatsuka T, Imabayashi E, Matsuda H, et al. Discrimination of dementia with Lewy bodies from Alzheimer's disease using voxel-based morphometry of white matter by statistical parametric mapping 8 plus diffeomorphic anatomic registration through exponentiated Lie algebra. Neuroradiology 2013;55(5):559–66.
51. Minoshima S, Foster NL, Sima AA, et al. Alzheimer's disease versus dementia with Lewy bodies: cerebral metabolic distinction with autopsy confirmation. Ann Neurol 2001;50(3):358–65.
52. Walker RW, Walker Z. Dopamine transporter single photon emission computerized tomography in the diagnosis of dementia with Lewy bodies. Mov Disord 2009;24(Suppl 2):S754–9.
53. Litvan I. Update on epidemiological aspects of progressive supranuclear palsy. Mov Disord 2003;18(Suppl 6):S43–50.
54. Lubarsky M, Juncos JL. Progressive supranuclear palsy: a current review. Neurologist 2008;14(2):79–88.
55. Liscic RM, Srulijes K, Groger A, et al. Differentiation of progressive supranuclear palsy: clinical, imaging and laboratory tools. Acta Neurol Scand 2013;127(5): 362–70.
56. Zhao P, Zhang B, Gao S. 18F-FDG PET study on the idiopathic Parkinson's disease from several parkinsonian-plus syndromes. Parkinsonism Relat Disord 2012;18(Suppl 1):S60–2.
57. Wenning GK, Litvan I, Jankovic J, et al. Natural history and survival of 14 patients with corticobasal degeneration confirmed at postmortem examination. J Neurol Neurosurg Psychiatry 1998;64(2):184–9.
58. Whitwell JL, Jack CR Jr, Boeve BF, et al. Imaging correlates of pathology in corticobasal syndrome. Neurology 2010;75(21):1879–87.
59. Hosaka K, Ishii K, Sakamoto S, et al. Voxel-based comparison of regional cerebral glucose metabolism between PSP and corticobasal degeneration. J Neurol Sci 2002;199(1–2):67–71.
60. Eckert T, Barnes A, Dhawan V, et al. FDG PET in the differential diagnosis of parkinsonian disorders. NeuroImage 2005;26(3):912–21.

61. Teune LK, Bartels AL, de Jong BM, et al. Typical cerebral metabolic patterns in neurodegenerative brain diseases. Mov Disord 2010;25(14):2395–404.
62. Josephs KA, Whitwell JL, Boeve BF, et al. Anatomical differences between CBS-corticobasal degeneration and CBS-Alzheimer's disease. Mov Disord 2010;25(9): 1246–52.
63. Aylward EH, Codori AM, Barta PE, et al. Basal ganglia volume and proximity to onset in presymptomatic Huntington disease. Arch Neurol 1996;53(12):1293–6.
64. Manyam BV, Walters AS, Narla KR. Bilateral striopallidodentate calcinosis: clinical characteristics of patients seen in a registry. Mov Disord 2001;16(2):258–64.
65. Baugh CM, Stamm JM, Riley DO, et al. Chronic traumatic encephalopathy: neuro-degeneration following repetitive concussive and subconcussive brain trauma. Brain Imaging Behav 2012;6(2):244–54.
66. Hebb AO, Cusimano MD. Idiopathic normal pressure hydrocephalus: a systematic review of diagnosis and outcome. Neurosurgery 2001;49(5):1166–84 [discussion: 1184–6].
67. Wicklund MR, Mokri B, Drubach DA, et al. Frontotemporal brain sagging syndrome: an SIH-like presentation mimicking FTD. Neurology 2011;76(16):1377–82.
68. Gascon-Bayarri J, Mana J, Martinez-Yelamos S, et al. Neurosarcoidosis: report of 30 cases and a literature survey. Eur J Intern Med 2011;22(6):e125–32.
69. Kuruppu DK, Matthews BR. Young-onset dementia. Semin Neurol 2013;33(4): 365–85.
70. Greco A, De Virgilio A, Gallo A, et al. Susac's syndrome—pathogenesis, clinical variants and treatment approaches. Autoimmun Rev 2014;13(8):814–21.
71. Takada LT, Geschwind MD. Prion diseases. Semin Neurol 2013;33:348–56.
72. Muayqil T, Gronseth G, Camicioli R. Evidence-based guideline: diagnostic accuracy of CSF 14-3-3 protein in sporadic Creutzfeldt-Jakob disease: report of the guideline development subcommittee of the American Academy of Neurology. Neurology 2012;79(14):1499–506.
73. Charness ME. Brain lesions in alcoholics. Alcohol Clin Exp Res 1993;17(1):2–11.
74. Lawn ND, Westmoreland BF, Kiely MJ, et al. Clinical, magnetic resonance imaging, and electroencephalographic findings in paraneoplastic limbic encephalitis. Mayo Clin Proc 2003;78(11):1363–8.
75. Valcour V, Paul R, Chiao S, et al. Screening for cognitive impairment in human immunodeficiency virus. Clin Infect Dis 2011;53(8):836–42.
76. Read PJ, Donovan B. Clinical aspects of adult syphilis. Intern Med J 2012;42(6): 614–20.

Genetic Testing and Counseling in the Diagnosis and Management of Young-Onset Dementias

Jill S. Goldman, MS, MPhil

KEYWORDS

- Genetic counseling • Predictive genetic testing • Presymptomatic testing protocol
- Huntington disease • Alzheimer disease • Frontotemporal degeneration • CADASIL
- Prion disease

KEY POINTS

- Young-onset dementias can be hereditary, multifactorial, or sporadic. The most common hereditary dementias include Alzheimer disease (AD), frontotemporal degeneration (FTD), Huntington disease (HD), the prion diseases, and CADASIL.
- Because disease symptoms can overlap, careful attainment of family history can assist with diagnosis and determining the likelihood of a genetic cause, and can direct genetic testing.
- The type of genetic testing depends on the confidence of the diagnosis, patient's and affected relatives' symptoms, and the number of disease genes.
- Whereas the prion diseases, HD, and CADASIL are single-gene disorders, familial AD and FTD have several causal genes and genetic risk factors.
- Single-gene, disease-specific gene panels, and large dementia panels are available. Genetic counseling should be given and informed consent must be obtained.
- Predictive testing should follow the Huntington disease protocol.

INTRODUCTION

The terms early onset and young-onset dementia refer to the group of progressive neurodegenerative diseases that commonly affect individuals before the age of

Disclosures Statement: P50 AG08702, NIH/NIA; CU08-7254 PDF Parkinson's Disease Foundation Research Center Grant; 1R01NS076837-01A1 NIH/NINDS; HDSA; P50 5P50HG007257-02 NIH/NH-GRI Center for Research on Ethical, Legal and Social Implications of Psychiatric, Neurologic and Behavioral Genetics; R01AG045390 NIH/NIA.
Taub Institute for Research on Alzheimer's Disease and the Aging Brain, Columbia University Medical Center, 630 West 168th Street, Box 16, New York, NY 10032, USA
E-mail address: jg2673@cumc.columbia.edu

Psychiatr Clin N Am 38 (2015) 295–308
http://dx.doi.org/10.1016/j.psc.2015.01.008
0193-953X/15/$ – see front matter © 2015 Elsevier Inc. All rights reserved.

Abbreviations	
AD	Alzheimer's disease
ALS	Amyotrophic lateral sclerosis
bvFTD	Behavioral variant FTD
CADASIL	Cerebral autosomal-dominant arteriopathy with subcortical infarcts and leukoencephalopathy
CJD	Creutzfeldt-Jakob disease
EOAD	Early onset Alzheimer's disease
FFI	Fatal familial insomnia
FTD	Frontotemporal degeneration
GSS	Gerstmann-Sträussler-Scheinker syndrome
HD	Huntington disease
vCJD	Variant CJD

60 years.[1] These same conditions also can affect people later in life. However, the earlier forms of these conditions are more likely to have a genetic cause. Some young-onset dementias are 100% genetic, whereas others may have inherited and sporadic forms. Additionally, although most genetic metabolic disorders are symptomatic in childhood, they also have adult-onset forms that include dementia, and are caused by mild mutations in the associated genes causing later onset and less severe symptoms.

Young-onset dementia can exist as a primarily cognitive state, or be part of a larger syndrome. The primary dementias can also present with other features, such as parkinsonism, chorea, ataxia, migraine, motor neuron disease, or psychiatric disorder. However, subtle cognitive dysfunction is usually an initial symptom (**Table 1**). Yet the diagnosis of young-onset dementia is often delayed because of misattribution of symptoms as psychiatric rather than neurodegenerative.[2] This delay can be detrimental not only to the patient, but also the family. Potentially a delay in proper diagnosis prevents families from seeking dementia care guidance, planning for the future, and participating in treatment trials. Additionally, a delayed diagnosis of a hereditary dementia can impact reproductive and life choices for all family members. This article concentrates on the most common forms of young-onset dementias that can present with psychiatric features: Alzheimer disease (AD), frontotemporal

Table 1
Categories of young-onset hereditary dementias

Hereditary Primary Dementias	Hereditary Movement Disorders with Dementia	Hereditary Metabolic Diseases with Dementia
Alzheimer disease	Huntington disease	Adult Tay-Sachs disease
Frontotemporal dementia	Spinocerebellar ataxias	Kufs disease
Prion diseases	Dentatorubral-pallidoluysian atrophy	Adrenoleukodystrophy
CADASIL		Metachromatic leukodystrophy
Lewy body dementia (rarely hereditary)	Parkinson dementia	Mitochondrial encephalopathy, lactic acidosis, and stroke-like episodes, and other mitochondrial diseases
Other vascular dementias	Neuroacanthocytosis	Krabbe disease
		Fabry disease
		Niemann-Pick type C disease
		Wilson disease
		Adult polyglucosan body disease
		Cerebrotendinous xanthomatosis

degeneration (FTD), Huntington disease (HD), cerebral autosomal-dominant arterio-pathy with subcortical infarcts and leukoencephalopathy (CADASIL), and prion dis-eases. Because diagnosis and treatment is discussed elsewhere in this issue, this article concentrates on symptomology, psychiatric features, and genetics. The prac-tice and protocol for determining a genetic cause for these disorders and the appro-priate counseling involved in the process are discussed.

Throughout this discussion, it is important to keep in mind that genetic testing for these disorders can be complicated by the overlap in clinical phenotype (**Table 2**). Thus, careful documentation of family history and a full neurologic evaluation are essential before ordering a genetic test. Additionally, genetic testing can be very expensive and is not always covered by insurance (because results do not usually affect clinical management). Therefore, the ordering clinician needs to assess each case to determine the most efficacious type of genetic testing.

YOUNG-ONSET DEMENTIA AND GENETICS
Alzheimer Disease

According to the Alzheimer's Association, there are approximately 250,000 people in the United States with early onset Alzheimer's disease (EOAD).[1] This group is more likely to have a genetic cause for their disease than the much more prevalent late-onset disease. One to five percent of all AD is autosomal dominant with by a three-generational family history of early-onset AD.[3–5] Early onset familial AD is caused by autosomal-dominant mutations in three genes: presenilin 1 (*PSEN1* on chromosome 14), presenilin 2 (*PSEN2* on chromosome 1), and the amyloid precursor protein gene (*APP* on chromosome 21.) Of these, *PSEN1* accounts for about half of all the autosomal-dominant cases, with *APP* being the second most common gene, and mu-tations in *PSEN2* being very rare. To date according to the Alzheimer Disease & Fronto-temporal Dementia Mutation Database (http://www.molgen.vib-ua.be/ADMutations), 33 different *APP* mutations have been reported in 90 families, 185 *PSEN1* mutations

Table 2 Genes associated with hereditary dementias		
Gene	**Disease**	**Lifetime Penetrance**
APP	AD	~100%
PSEN1	AD	~100%
PSEN2	AD	<100%
APOE	AD	Susceptibility factor
MAPT	FTD	~100%
GRN	FTD	Approaching 100% with age
C9ORF72	FTD/ALS	Probably 100%
TARDBP	FTD/ALS	n/a
FUS	FTD/ALS	<100%
CHMP2B	FTD	100%
VCP	IBMPFD	100% (but only 35% FTD)
HTT	HD	100%
PRNP	CJD/GSS/FFI	Most 100%, some less
NOTCH3	CADASIL	100%

Abbreviations: ALS, amyotrophic lateral sclerosis; CJD, Creutzfeldt–Jakob disease; FFI, fatal familial insomnia; GSS, Gerstmann-Sträussler-Scheinker syndrome; IBMFD, inclusion body myopathy with early onset Paget disease and frontotemporal dementia.

have been reported in 405 families, and 13 *PSEN2* mutations have been reported in 22 families. Whereas unaffected elderly carriers of *PSEN2* mutations have been reported, penetrance of *PSEN1* and *APP* mutations is thought to approach 100%.[6]

Onset of symptoms for *PSEN1* and *APP* mutations is typically in the fifth and sixth decades, and somewhat later for *PSEN2* mutations. However, onset with *PSEN1* mutations has been reported as early as the late 20s.[7] Additionally, onset can be variable even within families. Typical memory problems similar to those of late-onset AD are the most common presenting symptoms; however, behavioral change, mood disorder, and a dysexecutive syndrome frequently occur and can complicate diagnosis. Specific mutations in these genes can be associated with noncognitive features, such as cerebral amyloid angiopathy, spastic paraplegia, and seizures.[8]

In addition to these three autosomal-dominant genes, other genes, such as the apolipoprotein E gene (*APOE*) increase risk and the likelihood of seeing a family history of AD. *APOE* exists in three allelic forms: e2, e3, and e4. Having a single e4 allele increases the lifetime risk of developing AD two to four times over background risk reaching 50% if someone lives past age 80.[9] Having two copies of e4 increases risk to about 10 to 15 times that of the general population.[10] *APOE* e4 also lowers the average age of onset of symptoms.[10] Yet *APOE* e4 is neither necessary nor sufficient for developing AD, and overall risk depends on a combination of genetic, epigenetic, and environmental factors. Thus, current guidelines do not advocate testing for APOE status.[11] Ongoing genome-wide association studies and future whole exome/genome sequencing have and will identify many other risk genes.

Psychiatric aspects of young-onset Alzheimer disease

Insight is often cited as deficient in dementia; however, many individuals with EOAD may retain far more insight about their deficits than their later-onset counterparts. This greater awareness can be associated with dysthymia.[12] De Vliet and colleagues[12] emphasize that physicians can use their patients' increased awareness to help motivate them to participate in planning their future life plans and take care of financial issues.

Although studies have reported mixed results, a longitudinal study of patients with young-onset compared with late-onset AD demonstrated less neuropsychiatric symptoms in the younger group. The most common symptom in the younger group was apathy. Frontal variant AD may be another presentation in the EOAD population.[13] Behavioral/personality change may result in delayed diagnoses or misdiagnosis as psychiatric disorder or FTD. An awareness of family history of AD can be advantageous in early diagnosis.

Frontotemporal Degeneration

With an incidence of 2.7 to 4.1 per 100,000 people, FTD is one of the most common causes of young-onset dementia.[14] FTD presents with behavioral/personality changes (behavioral variant FTD [bvFTD]), or as primary progressive aphasia. Whereas language deficits are quickly identified as a neurologic condition, behavioral symptoms are frequently misattributed to psychiatric disorder, leading to psychiatrists being the point of entry to diagnosis. Criteria for bvFTD include at least three of the following[15]:

- Disinhibition
- Apathy or inertia
- Loss of empathy
- Perseverative
- Stereotyped or compulsive/ritualistic behavior

- Hyperorality and dietary change
- Executive/generation deficits with relative sparing of memory and visuospatial function

Because an individual with bvFTD generally lacks significant insight, an interview with an informant is essential to diagnosis.

A family history of FTD or a related neurodegenerative condition (AD, Parkinson disease, amyotrophic lateral sclerosis [ALS]) is found in 30% to 50% of cases. However, a true autosomal-dominant family history is far less common and accounts for about 10% of cases.[16] Three major and four much rarer genes have been associated with autosomal-dominant FTD (see **Table 2**). Mutations in *MAPT* (the tau gene) and *GRN* (the progranulin gene), and a hexanucleotide expansion (GGGGCC) in *C9orf72* are together responsible for between 60% and 80% of familial FTD. *C9orf72* is also the most common causal gene for familial ALS, and accounts for most families with both FTD and ALS in their histories. Other autosomal-dominant and risk alleles may still be unknown. Whereas *MAPT* seems to be 100% penetrant, a few elderly carriers of *GRN* mutations have been identified.[17] Recently, homozygous variants in *TMEM106B* have been found to be protective of FTD in *GRN* carriers. This same gene may protect *C9orf72* carriers from FTD but not ALS.[18] Additionally *GRN* and *C9orf72* mutations have been found in about 3% to 6% of sporadic FTD cases.[17,19,20]

Psychiatric aspects of frontotemporal degeneration

bvFTD presents with symptoms that are often confused with psychiatric disease.[21] When a patient with bvFTD presents to a psychiatrist, correct diagnosis may be complicated by the inability to interview a reliable informant. However, every attempt should be made to do so, because the patient may have little insight into his or her deficiencies. Treatment of psychiatric symptoms with selective serotonin reuptake inhibitors may abate some problems; however, the family may be misled about the cause of the symptoms, thus delaying necessary precautions and future planning. A thorough neurologic and neuropsychological assessment is essential for determining the actual cause of symptoms.

Additionally carriers of the *C9orf72* expansion may present with late-onset psychotic features including hallucinations and delusions. Carriers of the expansion can show psychiatric features in a prodromal period long before signs of dementia appear.[22,23] A careful neurologic and psychiatric family history may reveal the existence of an FTD-related disease.

Huntington Disease

HD is the prototypic autosomal-dominant neurodegenerative disease. The HD protocol for genetic testing is now the gold standard for all neurodegenerative conditions.[24,25] The prevalence of HD is 5 to 10 per 100,000 people in North and South America, Europe, and Australia, and lower prevalence in Asia and Africa.[26] Onset of symptoms can occur from childhood (juvenile HD) to late life but most typically is 30 to 50 years.[27] HD is considered a movement disorder and dementia. For many patients, it is also a psychiatric disease. HD is characterized by slowly progressive motor symptoms including chorea, dysarthria, eye movement abnormalities, incoordination, bradykinesia, rigidity, dystonia, and cognitive impairment including cognitive slowing, reduced attention, dysexecutive syndrome, and lack of insight.[27] The course of the disease varies considerably with cognitive symptoms proceeding or following onset of motor symptoms.

HD is caused by an expansion of the CAG tract of the *HTT* gene, and is thus known as a triple repeat disease or polyglutamine disease (because CAG codes for the amino acid glutamine). An inverse correlation of about 60% to 70% exists between the number of repeats and age of onset (**Table 3**).[28] The normal allele consists of 26 or fewer CAG repeats. Individuals with 40 or more repeats definitely develop HD. The repeat range between 36 and 39 (gray area) demonstrates reduced age-dependent penetrance so that some people become affected but usually at a later than the average age of onset. In this range, symptoms can be milder and progress more slowly.[26] The 26 to 35 repeat range, known as the intermediate allele range, was originally thought to be asymptomatic but meiotically unstable so that a germline expansion can occur causing earlier onset in the next generation. However, many studies have reported a behavioral/psychiatric phenotype without motor or cognitive symptoms. When compared with control subjects, the intermediate repeat group shows greater irritability, anxiety, depression, obsessive thinking, and apathy.[29]

The phenomenon of anticipation is found in HD whereby age of onset may decrease in each successive generation. Anticipation results from the germline expansion of an unstable allele. Expansion is much more likely to occur during paternal transmission than maternal. Very occasionally a small contraction occurs, usually when maternally transmitted.[26]

Psychiatric aspects of Huntington disease

Psychiatric features of HD are less consistent than motor symptoms. The most commonly seen symptoms are depression, irritability, anxiety, and apathy.[27,30] These symptoms should be treated appropriately. Additionally, psychiatric symptoms may be seen in people with intermediate and gray area repeat ranges. This last group is hard to detect because they usually lack a family history of HD. Additionally, these individuals may be at risk for adverse outcomes following predictive testing.[31] Thus, a careful assessment of mood and suicidal tendencies is required before testing. Lastly, children with juvenile HD may present with behavioral symptoms and cognitive impairment. Bradykinesia and dystonia are more common in juvenile HD than chorea.[32] A diagnosis of juvenile HD should be considered in children presenting with unexplained behavioral and cognitive changes with or without motor symptoms but with a positive family history of HD.

As with all hereditary neurodegenerative diseases, those at risk, particularly in the prodromal period, may experience significant depression and anxiety as they approach the age of onset of their parent.[33] Therapy and pharmacologic treatment can be beneficial. Suicidality is more common among gene carriers than noncarriers, and needs to be addressed with these patients.[34]

Prion Disease

The human prion diseases are caused by an accumulation of abnormal prion protein (PrP^{Sc}) in the brain. The prevalence of these diseases is 1 per 1,000,000. The most

Table 3
HTT CAG repeat ranges and phenotype

Number of CAG Repeats	Phenotype	Average Age of Onset
≤26	Normal	—
27–35	None or psychiatric	Late life if at all
36–39	None or HD	Late life
≥40	HD	30–50
≥50	Juvenile HD	<20

common form of the disease, Creutzfeldt-Jakob disease (CJD), is generally a very rapidly progressive dementia. Whereas most cases are sporadic, 10% to 15% of CJD is caused by mutations in the prion gene (*PRNP*). A second prion disease, Gerstmann-Sträussler-Scheinker syndrome (GSS), is always caused by mutations in *PRNP*, and a third form, fatal familial insomnia (FFI), is also almost always caused by mutation in this gene. All genetic forms of the disease demonstrate autosomal-dominant inheritance. The distinct phenotype is determined by the mutation, the genotype of a polymorphism at codon 129 (and probably that of other polymorphisms), and the physiochemical properties of PrP^{Sc}.[35] Codon 129 has two allelic forms that encode for either methionine (M) or valine (V). Being homozygous for either of these greatly increases the risk of sporadic CJD and the MM genotype has been found in all variant CJD (vCJD) associated with the mad cow disease outbreak. In genetic prion disease, the combination of a specific mutation and its chromosome-associated (*cis*) codon 129 allele influences the phenotype, age of onset, and disease duration. For example, the D178N mutation with *cis* M results in FFI, whereas with V, the phenotype is that of CJD. The genotype of the other allele may further influence onset and duration.[36] Because of the polymorphism influence, phenotype is variable within and among families.

More than 30 *PRNP* mutations have been reported. Most of these are single nucleotide changes. However, there is an octapeptide repeat sequence that, when altered in number of repeats, results in CJD with much longer duration and an onset with psychiatric/behavioral and cognitive disturbances. Although most mutations seem to be close to 100% penetrant, some demonstrate reduced penetrance. Reduced penetrance may be responsible for part of the 60% of familial cases without a family history.[37] A lack of family history may also be caused by lost information, misdiagnoses, early death, undeclared adoption, false paternity, or the possibility of *de novo* mutations. Specific mutations result in the FFI and GSS phenotypes.

CJD often begins with a psychiatric profile of depression, anxiety, and agitation. This is especially true of vCJD and with younger onset in general.[38] The mean age of onset for vCJD is 27 and duration is about 14 months. Sporadic CJD presents with cognitive impairment including memory, executive, or language dysfunction in 40% of cases. Other common early symptoms include cerebellar signs, headaches, dizziness, sleep disorder, and visual abnormalities. As the disease progresses, these symptoms worsen and parkinsonism, dystonia, myoclonus, and seizures become common additional features.[39] The mean age of onset for sporadic CJD is about 68 with a large range of ages, and the mean duration is 7 months. Inherited CJD is variable in age of onset, duration, and clinical symptoms depending on the *PRNP* mutation and the allelic variants at codon 129 of the gene. In addition to the symptoms listed previously, neuropathy may be an early feature of genetic CJD.

FFI generally begins with insomnia and sleep disturbances and progresses to dementia, mood disorder, dysarthria, ataxia, and myoclonus.[35] Duration is about 15 months.[39] GSS usually presents as a movement disorder with ataxia or parkinsonism. Slow cognitive decline follows. The disease has a long duration of 3 to 8 years.[39]

Psychiatric aspects of prion diseases
The prion disease may begin with behavioral or mood changes. A sudden onset of symptoms may be a red flag for considering prion disease. Agitation and irritability are the most common presenting symptoms that occur before the onset of physical symptoms. Furthermore, disinhibition, impulsivity, and depression may be seen. Early psychiatric symptoms are particularly prominent in vCJD.[38] A sudden onset of

psychiatric symptoms should warrant a neurologic evaluation. Agitation and psychosis (including hallucinations) is common during disease progression.

Cerebral Autosomal-Dominant Arteriopathy with Subcortical Infarcts and Leukoencephalopathy

CADASIL is a rare disease (prevalence of ~4 per 100,000 people)[40] yet the most common cause of inherited stroke, particularly in younger adults. CADASIL is caused by autosomal-dominant mutations in the *NOTCH3* gene. Mutations cause recurrent subcortical ischemic strokes resulting in mood and personality change, gradually progressive cognitive impairment and eventual dementia, and motor disturbances. In 20% to 40% of people, migraine with aura is a precursor to cognitive changes.[40] Seizures occur in 5% to 10% of patients. The mean age of onset for the first ischemic event is about 50, but the range of onset is large. Mean disease duration is approximately 25 years. Although variable in presentation and onset, CADASIL is thought to have near complete lifetime penetrance.[41]

Psychiatric aspects of cerebral autosomal-dominant arteriopathy with subcortical infarcts and leukoencephalopathy

Depression is a common early symptom of CADASIL and may present before the onset of overt neurologic symptoms. CADASIL should be suspected in the presence of a history of migraine with aura, cognitive decline (particularly executive function dysfunction), or a positive family history of stroke with or without migraines. In addition to depression, emotional lability, anger, apathy, and bipolar-like disorder have been reported.[42–44] In some cases, psychiatric symptoms are intractable despite medication.[45]

GENETIC COUNSELING AND TESTING FOR INHERITED DEMENTIAS

Genetic counseling should always precede genetic testing to allow the patient and family to understand the possibility of a genetic cause and the resultant risk to other family members. Genetic counseling can be done by a well-informed physician or genetic counselor (see www.nsgc.org to find a counselor in your area). Either should be well-versed in the genetics of dementia.

One of the best tools for clues to diagnosis is a thorough three-generation pedigree. Any history of a neurologic or psychiatric condition should be carefully explored. If possible, age of onset of symptoms, the nature of the first symptom, and date of death should be explored in each affected relative. Patients with their informant should be asked about the patient's siblings, parents, aunts and uncles, first cousins, grandparents, and great aunts and uncles. Specific questions generate much more information than more general ones (**Box 1**). An example of how the pedigree will help is, hearing that a family member died of ALS might guide the clinician toward FTD and a *C9orf72* mutation, or hearing about a rapidly progressive disease might point to hereditary CJD.

If a genetic disorder is suspected, a complete neurologic evaluation is necessary to further narrow the differential diagnosis. At that point, genetic testing may be ordered to confirm diagnosis or to give more information to the family. However, genetic counseling and informed consent are essential before ordering any genetic test so that the patient and family fully understand the implications for other family members (**Box 2**). It is important to remember that not all families want this information. Of particular importance is a discussion of all possible test results including the possibility of a variant of unknown significance. If a variant of unknown significance is found, not only will it be unclear whether the disease is genetic, but other family members will be unable to do predictive testing.

Box 1
Family history questions

Has anyone had cognitive impairment including memory loss or dementia?

Has anyone had behavioral or personality changes?

Has anyone had trouble with language or speaking?

Has anyone had depression, bipolar disease, or psychotic events?

Has anyone had migraines?

Has anyone had strokes or stroke-like events?

Has anyone had seizures?

Has anyone had a neurologic disease, such as ALS or Parkinson disease?

Has anyone had trouble walking?

Has anyone had jerky movements or tremor?

Several types of diagnostic genetic tests are available. These include single-gene sequencing, which is appropriate when the diagnosis is certain (as for HD), a disease-specific gene panel when more than one gene can cause the disease (AD, FTD), or a larger gene panel when several diagnoses are being considered (dementia panel by next-generation sequencing). Whole exome or genome testing is not advised because most dementia genes are covered by the previously mentioned tests and whole exome/genome sequencing generates large numbers of variants of unknown significance and secondary findings that might reveal the risk for other diseases.

Predictive Testing for Young-Onset Dementia

Once a mutation has been discovered in an affected person, other family members might want to explore predictive testing. Predictive testing should not be ordered on demand. Instead, predictive testing requires significant work, contemplation, and

---

Box 2
Topics for the genetic counseling discussion concerning diagnostic genetic testing

Nature of suspected diagnosis and why it is being considered

Review of family history

Previous experience with the disease in the family

Autosomal-dominant inheritance and 50% risk to first-degree relatives

Penetrance of gene

What the genetic test is looking for (point mutation, repeat expansion, duplication/deletion, and so forth)

Possible results (positive, negative, variant of unknown significance, repeat range)

Any anticipation in next generation

Whether results will be communicated to family members and how

Possibility of predictive testing for family members

Available resources for disease (support groups, research, and so forth)

care as suggested by the HD protocol. The HD protocol was established as a systematic way to provide time for careful thought by and evaluation of the patient before embarking on testing to avert negative outcomes.[24,25] Studies show that only about 18% of at-risk relatives elect to have predictive testing. These individuals are self-selected and usually go through the rigorous protocol, yet some at-risk individuals who present to a predictive testing program drop out before testing. Of those who complete testing, about 17% have a serious adverse effect, such as depression or significant psychological distress, although most express beneficial outcomes.[46,47]

The HD protocol (**Fig. 1**) is extensive and time consuming for the patient. Although it is stressful, the prolonged consideration of the implication of testing results in some patients choosing to forego testing. Others are directed to therapy to develop better coping strategies for anxiety or depression before the possibility of a positive (CAG expansion) result.

The protocol has been criticized for being paternalistic. As a result, the World Congress on Huntington Disease will review the new 2012 guidelines[25] every 2 years. Regardless, the existing guidelines have provided a framework for assessing patients and providing a case-by-case adaptation to the guidelines.

Guidelines on genetic testing for adult-onset diseases including dementia strongly recommend that minors not be tested until they reach an age to make an informed

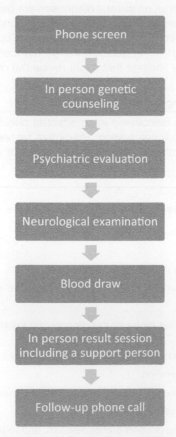

Fig. 1. The Huntington disease protocol for predictive testing.

decision. However, special cases may arise in which testing is in the best interest of the child. In these situations, the minor's assent and the parent's consent should be obtained (Position Statement on Genetic Testing of Minors for Adult-Onset Conditions http://nsgc.org/p/bl/ar/blogaid=28).[48,49]

Whether or not they provide initial genetic counseling, psychiatrists can be an excellent resource for people undergoing predictive testing. The psychiatrist can help the patient examine the potential impact of a positive result through anticipatory guidance, and also help them assess their own ability to cope with an adverse outcome, including survivor guilt generated by a negative result. Patients should examine their extended circle of support within and outside the immediate family. Additionally, the psychiatrist is essential to the process of assessing whether the patient is ready to undergo predictive testing or should be bolstered by additional therapy and/or medication.

SUMMARY

Young-onset dementia can ravage not only the affected individual, but also the family. This is especially true when the cause of the disease is genetic. Early diagnosis and appropriate treatment is essential to establishing a manageable quality of life for patient and caregiver. Genetic counseling provides information on possible disease cause and the mechanism behind that cause. Through analysis of past family experience and anticipatory guidance, the patient and family can assess whether learning of a genetic cause will be helpful or harmful. This is especially true of predictive testing. Genetic testing requires a careful assessment of the implications of a positive and negative test. Finding a mutation in a person affected with a dementia informs risk to others. Whether and how this risk is conveyed is an essential part of pretest and posttest counseling. Predictive testing can reduce anxiety caused by uncertainty and provide information for life and reproductive choices. However, without proper preparation and support, predictive testing can cause depression and more anxiety. Psychiatric assessment is necessary before testing occurs to help determine the risk of adverse outcomes for the individual. Additionally, the outcome can be improved by psychiatric support during and after the testing.

Genetic testing is a powerful tool for facilitating diagnosis of young-onset dementia. As gene-specific drug trials come to fruition, access to genetic testing will become even more important. Genetic counseling and psychiatric support are invaluable for patients and families during this process.

REFERENCES

1. Thies W, Bleiler L, Alzheimer's A. 2013 Alzheimer's disease facts and figures. Alzheimers Dement 2013;9:208–45.
2. van Vliet D, de Vugt ME, Bakker C, et al. Time to diagnosis in young-onset dementia as compared with late-onset dementia. Psychol Med 2013;43:423–32.
3. Jiang T, Yu JT, Tian Y, et al. Epidemiology and etiology of Alzheimer's disease: from genetic to non-genetic factors. Curr Alzheimer Res 2013;10:852–67.
4. Bertram L, Tanzi RE. The genetics of Alzheimer's disease. Prog Mol Biol Transl Sci 2012;107:79–100.
5. Bekris LM, Yu CE, Bird TD, et al. Genetics of Alzheimer disease. J Geriatry Psychiatry Neurol 2010;23:213–27.
6. Tanzi RE. The genetics of Alzheimer disease. Cold Spring Harb Perspect Med 2012;2:a006296.

7. Larner AJ. Frontal variant Alzheimer's disease: a reappraisal. Clin Neurol Neurosurg 2006;108:705–8.
8. Alonso Vilatela ME, Lopez-Lopez M, Yescas-Gomez P. Genetics of Alzheimer's disease. Arch Med Res 2012;43:622–31.
9. Ringman JM, Coppola G. New genes and new insights from old genes: update on Alzheimer disease. Continuum 2013;19:358–71.
10. Slooter AJ, Cruts M, Kalmijn S, et al. Risk estimates of dementia by apolipoprotein E genotypes from a population-based incidence study: the Rotterdam Study. Arch Neurol 1998;55:964–8.
11. Goldman JS, Hahn SE, Catania JW, et al. Genetic counseling and testing for Alzheimer disease: joint practice guidelines of the American college of medical genetics and the national society of genetic counselors. Genet Med 2011;13:597–605.
12. van Vliet D, de Vugt ME, Kohler S, et al. Awareness and its association with affective symptoms in young-onset and late-onset Alzheimer disease: a prospective study. Alzheimer Dis Assoc Disord 2013;27:265–71.
13. Nygaard HB, Lippa CF, Mehdi D, et al. A novel presenilin 1 mutation in early-onset Alzheimer's disease with prominent frontal features. Am J Alzheimers Dis Other Demen 2014;29:433–5.
14. Onyike CU, Diehl-Schmid J. The epidemiology of frontotemporal dementia. Int Rev Psychiatry 2013;25:130–7.
15. Rascovsky K, Hodges JR, Knopman D, et al. Sensitivity of revised diagnostic criteria for the behavioural variant of frontotemporal dementia. Brain 2011;134:2456–77.
16. Rohrer JD, Guerreiro R, Vandrovcova J, et al. The heritability and genetics of frontotemporal lobar degeneration. Neurology 2009;73:1451–6.
17. Le Ber I, van der Zee J, Hannequin D, et al. Progranulin null mutations in both sporadic and familial frontotemporal dementia. Hum Mutat 2007;28:846–55.
18. van Blitterswijk M, Mullen B, Nicholson AM, et al. TMEM106B protects C9ORF72 expansion carriers against frontotemporal dementia. Acta Neuropathol 2014;127:397–406.
19. Majounie E, Abramzon Y, Renton AE, et al. Repeat expansion in C9ORF72 in Alzheimer's disease. N Engl J Med 2012;366:283–4.
20. DeJesus-Hernandez M, Mackenzie IR, Boeve BF, et al. Expanded GGGGCC hexanucleotide repeat in noncoding region of C9ORF72 causes chromosome 9p-linked FTD and ALS. Neuron 2011;72:245–56.
21. Mendez MF, Shapira JS, McMurtray A, et al. Accuracy of the clinical evaluation for frontotemporal dementia. Arch Neurol 2007;64:830–5.
22. Devenney E, Hornberger M, Irish M, et al. Frontotemporal dementia associated with the C9ORF72 mutation: a unique clinical profile. JAMA Neurol 2014;71:331–9.
23. Galimberti D, Fenoglio C, Serpente M, et al. Autosomal dominant frontotemporal lobar degeneration due to the C9ORF72 hexanucleotide repeat expansion: late-onset psychotic clinical presentation. Biol Psychiatry 2013;74:384–91.
24. Guidelines for the molecular genetics predictive test in Huntington's disease. International Huntington association (IHA) and the World federation of neurology (WFN) research group on Huntington's chorea. Neurology 1994;44:1533–6.
25. MacLeod R, Tibben A, Frontali M, et al. Recommendations for the predictive genetic test in Huntington's disease. Clin Genet 2013;83:221–31.

26. Reiner A, Dragatsis I, Dietrich P. Genetics and neuropathology of Huntington's disease. Int Rev Neurobiol 2011;98:325–72.
27. Ross CA, Aylward EH, Wild EJ, et al. Huntington disease: natural history, biomarkers and prospects for therapeutics. Nat Rev Neurol 2014;10:204–16.
28. Gusella JF, MacDonald ME. Huntington's disease: the case for genetic modifiers. Genome Med 2009;1:80.
29. Killoran A, Biglan KM, Jankovic J, et al. Characterization of the Huntington intermediate CAG repeat expansion phenotype in PHAROS. Neurology 2013;80: 2022–7.
30. van Duijn E, Kingma EM, van der Mast RC. Psychopathology in verified Huntington's disease gene carriers. J Neuropsychiatry Clin Neurosci 2007;19: 441–8.
31. Semaka A, Hayden MR. Evidence-based genetic counselling implications for Huntington disease intermediate allele predictive test results. Clin Genet 2014; 85:303–11.
32. Roos RA. Huntington's disease: a clinical review. Orphanet J Rare Dis 2010;5:40.
33. Epping EA, Mills JA, Beglinger LJ, et al. Characterization of depression in prodromal Huntington disease in the neurobiological predictors of HD (PREDICT-HD) study. J Psychiatr Res 2013;47:1423–31.
34. Hubers AA, van Duijn E, Roos RA, et al. Suicidal ideation in a European Huntington's disease population. J Affect Disord 2013;151:248–58.
35. Capellari S, Strammiello R, Saverioni D, et al. Genetic Creutzfeldt-Jakob disease and fatal familial insomnia: insights into phenotypic variability and disease pathogenesis. Acta Neuropathol 2011;121:21–37.
36. Gambetti P, Kong Q, Zou W, et al. Sporadic and familial CJD: classification and characterisation. Br Med Bull 2003;66:213–39.
37. Kovacs GG, Puopolo M, Ladogana A, et al. Genetic prion disease: the EUROCJD experience. Hum Genet 2005;118:166–74.
38. Thompson A, MacKay A, Rudge P, et al. Behavioral and psychiatric symptoms in prion disease. Am J Psychiatry 2014;171:265–74.
39. Takada LT, Geschwind MD. Prion diseases. Semin Neurol 2013;33:348–56.
40. Chabriat H, Joutel A, Dichgans M, et al. Cadasil. Lancet Neurol 2009;8: 643–53.
41. Sabbadini G, Francia A, Calandriello L, et al. Cerebral autosomal dominant arteriopathy with subcortical infarcts and leucoencephalopathy (CADASIL). Clinical, neuroimaging, pathological and genetic study of a large Italian family. Brain 1995; 118(Pt 1):207–15.
42. Noh SM, Chung SJ, Kim KK, et al. Emotional disturbance in CADASIL: its impact on quality of life and caregiver burden. Cerebrovasc Dis 2014;37:188–94.
43. Park S, Park B, Koh MK, et al. Case report: bipolar disorder as the first manifestation of CADASIL. BMC Psychiatry 2014;14:175.
44. Reyes S, Viswanathan A, Godin O, et al. Apathy: a major symptom in CADASIL. Neurology 2009;72:905–10.
45. Chabriat H, Bousser MG. Neuropsychiatric manifestations in CADASIL. Dialogues Clin Neurosci 2007;9:199–208.
46. Wedderburn S, Panegyres PK, Andrew S, et al. Predictive gene testing for Huntington disease and other neurodegenerative disorders. Intern Med J 2013;43: 1272–9.
47. Paulsen JS, Nance M, Kim JI, et al. A review of quality of life after predictive testing for and earlier identification of neurodegenerative diseases. Prog Neurobiol 2013;110:2–28.

48. European Society of Human Genetics. Genetic testing in asymptomatic minors: recommendations of the European Society of Human Genetics. Eur J Hum Genet 2009;17:720–1.
49. Ross LF, Saal HM, David KL, et al. Technical report: ethical and policy issues in genetic testing and screening of children. Genet Med 2013;15:234–45.

The Use of Cerebrospinal Fluid and Neuropathologic Studies in Neuropsychiatry Practice and Research

Kalyani Kansal, MBBS[a], David J. Irwin, MD[b],*

KEYWORDS

- CSF • Biomarkers • Neurodegenerative disease • Frontotemporal dementia • Prion
- Alzheimer disease • Parkinson disease • Dementia with Lewy bodies

KEY POINTS

- Currently there is no way to definitively diagnose neurodegenerative diseases (ie, Alzheimer disease [AD]; Parkinson disease [PD]; dementia with Lewy bodies [DLB]; frontotemporal dementia [FTD]; amyotrophic lateral sclerosis [ALS]) before neuropathologic examination at autopsy.
- The lack of specific tests (biomarkers) for neurodegenerative diseases necessitates a strategy of exclusion of infectious, neuroinflammatory, toxic, and other nonneurodegenerative etiologies (eg, rapidly progressive dementias [RPD]) that can mimic these conditions.
- Cerebrospinal fluid (CSF) analysis provides an important method for excluding RPD in the diagnostic evaluation for patients with suspected neurodegenerative conditions. Cerebral biopsy may be useful in select clinical scenarios.
- Detection of key pathologic proteins in the CSF in research studies of patients with AD, PD, DLB, FTD and ALS may provide critical biomarkers to improve diagnosis of these conditions during life. Validation efforts are currently underway to help bring these evaluations to clinical practice.

INTRODUCTION

Neurodegenerative disease encompasses a range of cognitive and motor features that are frequently encountered in neuropsychiatric practice, such as Alzheimer disease (AD), Parkinson disease (PD), dementia with Lewy bodies (DLB), frontotemporal

Disclosure: Support for this work was provided by grants from the National Institutes of Health (K23NS088341-01) and Jane Tanger Black Fund for Young-Onset Dementia.
[a] Department of Psychiatry and Behavioral Sciences, Johns Hopkins University School of Medicine, 550 North Broadway, Suite 305, Baltimore, MD 21205, USA; [b] Department of Neurology, Hospital of the University of Pennsylvania, University of Pennsylvania Perelman School of Medicine, 3 Gates, 3400 Spruce Street, Philadelphia, PA 19104, USA
* Corresponding author.
E-mail address: dirwin@mail.med.upenn.edu

Abbreviations	
AD	Alzheimer disease
ALS	Amyotrophic lateral sclerosis
CJD	Creutzfeldt-Jakob disease
CNS	Central nervous system
CSF	Cerebrospinal fluid
DLB	Dementia with Lewy bodies
FTD	Frontotemporal dementia
HE	Hashimoto encephalopathy
HIV	Human immunodeficiency virus
HSV-1	Herpes simplex virus-1
PCNSL	Primary CNS lymphoma
PCR	Polymerase chain reaction
PD	Parkinson disease
PrP	Prion protein
p-tau	Phosphorylated-tau
RPD	Rapidly progressive dementia
t-tau	Total-tau

dementia (FTD), and amyotrophic lateral sclerosis (ALS). A major limitation is the inability to confirm the diagnosis until neuropathologic examination at autopsy. Furthermore, metabolic conditions, such as vitamin B_{12} deficiency or hypothyroidism, are associated with cognitive deficits that may be easily confused for an early stage of a neurodegenerative condition. In particular, rapidly progressive dementias (RPDs) comprise a broad range of differential diagnoses (**Table 1**) that can mimic early symptoms of neurodegenerative disease. For a comprehensive overview and diagnostic/therapeutic algorithms of these conditions, see the article by Paterson and colleagues.[1] Clues of a nonneurodegenerative disease mimic or RPD include sudden-onset, stepwise, or rapid progression of symptoms; seizures; and neuroimaging

Table 1
Differential diagnosis of potential mimics of neurodegenerative disease

Category	Examples
Vascular	Infarct-related, primary/secondary CNS vasculitis, venous sinus thrombosis
Autoimmune	Hashimoto encephalopathy (steroid-responsive encephalopathy), paraneoplastic limbic encephalitis, neurosarcoidosis, demyelinating disease (eg, acute demyelinating encephalomyelitis), celiac sprue, neuropsychiatric systemic lupus erythematosus
Neoplastic	Primary/secondary CNS lymphoma, primary brain neoplasm, CNS/leptomeninges metastases
Infectious	Herpes simplex, *Treponema pallidum*, *Borrelia burgdorferi*, *Tropheryma whipplei*, *Cryptococcus neoformans*, HIV, progressive multifocal leukoencephalopathy
Prion disease	Creutzfeldt-Jakob disease
Toxic-metabolic	Heavy metal intoxication (eg, lead, mercury, arsenic), vitamin deficiencies (B_{12}, thiamine), medication-related, end-stage liver disease, pontine/extrapontine central myelinolysis, inborn errors of metabolism (eg, acute intermittent porphyria, adult-onset leukodystrophies, mitochondrial disease), hypo/hyperthyroidism
Epileptic	Nonconvulsive status epilepticus (various underlying etiologies)

Abbreviation: CNS, central nervous system.

findings of white-matter hyperintensities, gadolinium enhancement, or diffusion-weighted abnormalities. Furthermore, careful review of medication lists is critical, because geriatric patients can be very sensitive to many common psychotropic drugs (eg, benzodiazepines, neuroleptics) resulting in fluctuating cognitive impairment. Finally, attention to systemic disease, such as pulmonary, renal, and liver status, is also important to rule out metabolic conditions that can mimic a neurodegenerative condition. For example, a history of rapid correction of hyponatremia should raise suspicion of central myelinolysis, whereas focal neurologic findings and seizures in a patient with known malignancy may indicate central metastasis. Neuroimaging studies can help confirm these etiologies and direct further laboratory testing. It is also important to rule out nonconvulsive status epilepticus with an electroencephalogram (EEG) in patients with encephalopathy at high risk of having seizure.

Although clinical diagnosis for these conditions relies on a comprehensive evaluation (ie, detailed history, physical examination, radiologic testing, blood and urine analysis, cerebrospinal fluid [CSF] analysis, biopsy, EEG and other ancillary testing) the focus of this article is on the use of CSF testing and biopsy for diagnosis of RPD and differentiation from neurodegenerative conditions. Early accurate diagnosis of neurodegenerative disease is critical, because many forms of RPDs are reversible if treatment is initiated at an early stage. Furthermore, early implementation of proper pharmacologic treatments (ie, acetylcholinesterase inhibitors for AD, dopaminergic agents for PD) and supportive care may improve quality of life and preserve life participation in neurodegenerative conditions. Finally, there has been a period of rapid growth in neurodegenerative disease research with improved knowledge of the underlying pathophysiology and natural history of these conditions in the past decade. In particular, CSF analysis has emerged as a source for several potential biomarkers to improve diagnosis of AD, PD, DLB, FTD, and ALS. This article also highlights current CSF biomarker research in neurodegenerative disease.

CEREBROSPINAL FLUID TESTING FOR RAPIDLY PROGRESSIVE DEMENTIAS

A lumbar puncture is helpful in identifying cases of nonneurodegenerative disease associated cognitive and/or motor decline, including RPDs. Routine clinical CSF testing consists of cell count; protein levels; oligoclonal bands; IgG index; and bacterial, fungal, and mycobacterial stains with culture. Elevations in CSF protein reflect inflammation and loss of blood-brain barrier function, whereas CSF cell counts and differential identify infiltration of immune cells in the central nervous system (CNS). Both cells and protein are elevated in a range of inflammatory, infectious, or neoplastic conditions and abnormalities in these screening tests can be helpful to direct further testing for specific causes including bacterial-specific serologies (eg, syphilis, Lyme disease), autoantibodies in serum/CSF (ie, paraneoplastic syndromes), viral/bacterial DNA polymerase chain reaction (PCR) (eg, viral encephalitis, Whipple disease), and flow cytometry (ie, primary or secondary CNS lymphoma)[1] as outlined later.

Vasculitides/Autoimmune/Paraneoplastic

CSF pleocytosis and elevated protein are often seen in several of the CNS vasculitides, infections, autoimmune, and neoplastic disorders, although presence of neither is mandatory.[1,2] Headaches, focal neurologic signs, and neuroimaging abnormalities consistent with stroke should raise suspicion of autoimmune CNS vasculitis and CSF abnormalities are found in 80% to 90% of patients.[3] Among vascular conditions, cerebral venous sinus thrombosis is often associated with a normal CSF[1] and suspected in patients with hypercoaguble risk factors. Finally, systemic vasculitides can also affect the CNS (for a review see Berlit[4]).

In case of autoimmune disease, diagnosis is typically by detection of autoanti-bodies. In Hashimoto encephalopathy (HE or steroid-responsive encephalopathy), antithyroperoxidase and antithyroglobulin antibodies are elevated in CSF and serum.[5,6] For diagnosis of HE, other causes of RPD need to be ruled out in addition to detection of antibodies, because levels of antithyroid antibodies are elevated in 10% of the general population.[7] Systemic lupus erythematosus can involve the CNS and cause a range of neuropsychiatric symptoms including seizures, stroke, move-ment disorder, and diffuse encephalopathy, which is often associated with elevations of CSF protein and intrathecal IgG production, including antineuronal autoantibodies.[8] Other autoimmune conditions causing RPD include antiglutamic acid decarboxylase antibody syndrome and gluten-sensitivity dementia (celiac sprue), both of which may have detectable antibodies in the CSF or serum.[6,7] Most neurosarcoidosis cases have elevated CSF protein and pleocytosis, whereas increased CSF angiotensin-converting enzyme is less specific.[6] Clinical signs of pulmonary sarcoidosis, leptome-ningeal enhancement on MRI, and multiple cranial neuropathies (including optic neuritis) may raise the clinical suspicion of neurosarcoid.[9] Oligoclonal bands (ie, CSF immunoglobulins not found in serum) and increased IgG are other nonsensitive and nonspecific CSF markers associated with several immunologically mediated en-cephalopathies.[7,10] Neuroimaging findings of demyelination are helpful to identify those with multiple sclerosis, acute disseminated encephalomyelitis, and other auto-immune demyelinating disorders.

Among paraneoplastic limbic encephalitides, encephalopathy caused by voltage-gated VGKC antibodies is frequently associated with normal cell count and protein levels in the CSF.[10,11] Paraneoplastic limbic encephalitis is confirmed by detection of autoantibodies in CSF or serum, such as anti-Hu, anti-Ma2, anti-CV2, antiamphi-physin, anti-Zic4, anti-Ri, anti-VGKC, anti-NMDAR, and anti-AMPAR.[7] However, for some syndromes there is increased sensitivity for either CSF or serum testing. Indeed, anti-VGKC antibodies (frequently not associated with tumors) can be detected with greater sensitivity in the serum than in CSF.[11] However, in case of encephalopathy associated with anti-NMDAR antibodies, CSF has a higher antibody concentration than serum (suggesting an intrathecal synthesis of antibodies) and should be prefer-entially tested.[12] Similarly, anti-AMPAR antibodies should be tested for in CSF.[7] The cell surface antibodies (anti-VGKC, anti-NMDAR, anti-AMPAR) are associated with a better prognosis than the antibodies targeted at intraneuronal antigens (anti-Hu, anti-Ma2, anti-CV2, and so forth).[6] Clinically these patients may have a range of symp-toms including neuropsychiatric symptoms, seizures, autonomic instability, ataxia, headache, and a fluctuating course. Furthermore, a paraneoplastic syndrome frequently precedes the detection of a tumor, and presence of these antibodies must be followed by an aggressive search for the underlying tumor (**Table 2**) through detailed clinical assessment and imaging studies. If no malignancy is identified, clinical and radiographic surveillance should be repeated every 3 to 6 months for 2 to 3 years.[13]

Neoplastic

Among the neoplastic causes of RPD is primary CNS lymphoma (PCNSL), sometimes having a diffusely infiltrative pathology. CSF cytology is often negative in PCNSL[6] and flow cytometry has been recommended for lymphoma cells,[1] although it may also be negative.[14] Secondary involvement of the CNS by hematologic malignancies also may occur and can be detected by CSF flow cytometry. CNS tumors often are associated with elevated CSF protein and dural/meningeal metastasis can be identified by CSF cytology but lumbar punctures should be carefully considered because of the risk

Table 2
Cancers associated with paraneoplastic antibodies implicated in limbic encephalitis

Antibody	Commonly Associated Tumors
Against intracellular antigens	
Anti-Hu	SCLC
Anti-Ma2	Testicular germ-cell tumors, non-SCLC, breast cancer
Anti-CV2	SCLC, thymoma
Anti-Ri	Neuroblastoma in children, breast and ovary cancer in adults
Anti-amphiphysin	SCLC, breast cancer
Anti-Zic4	SCLC
Against cell membrane antigens	
Anti-VGKC	Thymoma, SCLC
Anti-NMDAR	Ovarian teratoma
Anti-AMPAR	Tumors of lung, breast, thymus

Abbreviation: SCLC, small cell lung cancer.

of herniation depending on the size, location, and mass effect of lesion on neuroimaging. Thus, it is necessary, especially when there is suspicion of a neoplasm or mass lesion, to obtain neuroimaging before performing a lumbar puncture.

Infectious

An important aspect of differential diagnosis for neurodegenerative disease mimics is the immune status of patients. Indeed, immunocompromised patients are at much higher risks of atypical opportunistic infections. Human immunodeficiency virus (HIV) itself can cause a range of cognitive impairment and motor disturbances (ie, HIV-associated neurocognitive disorders [HAND]).[15] As such, CSF analysis for bacterial, mycobacterial, and fungal culture and staining for infectious diseases[2] is critical for the evaluation of an unexplained mental status change in an immunocompromised patient.

Disease-specific serologies in CSF include VDRL for syphilis and intrathecal antibody production for *Borrelia burgdorferi* in CNS Lyme disease. The capsular antigen for *Cryptococcus neoformans* can be detected in CSF or visualized by India ink preparations.

PCR is another useful diagnostic technique. Indeed, estimation of viral loads of HIV in CSF correlates with cognitive impairment in HAND.[15] Reactivation of latent viral infections, such as human herpes virus-6 and JC virus (progressive multifocal leukoencephalopathy), can be detected by CSF PCR[16,17] and should be considered in patients with HIV or patients with solid/hematopoietic transplant with altered mental status and focal neurologic deficits. There are numerous other viral entities that can cause an acute infectious encephalopathy and CSF PCR and/or serologies for specific agents are essential, because viral culture can take several days to obtain.[18] Sensitivity of PCR for diagnosis of herpes simplex virus-1 (HSV-1) encephalitis is more than 90% and specificity is around 98%, although results may be negative within the first 72 hours of symptom onset.[10] HSV-1 encephalitis is also associated with a hemorrhagic necrosis that can be detected by persistent elevation in CSF red blood count. Finally, PCR and electron-microscopy have been used for detection of *Tropheryma whipplei* (causing Whipple disease) in the CSF.[6,19]

Prion Disease

One of the most devastating causes of RPD is the invariably fatal Creutzfeldt-Jakob disease (CJD), which is caused by an infectious protein particle (ie, prion protein

[PrP]). Most human cases are sporadic, whereas small subsets of cases are familial or associated with exposure to infected CNS tissue (ie, historical cadaveric human growth hormone epidemic, dural grafts, and so forth). CSF cells/protein are often normal in CJD, although mild pleocytosis may occur.[1] As such, increased CSF levels of 14-3-3, total-tau (t-tau), and neuron-specific enolase have been used as biomarkers for CJD, because CSF concentrations of these proteins are highly elevated as a consequence of the rapid neuronal damage seen in CJD. Diagnostic criteria for CJD includes CSF protein 14-3-3[20,21]; however, a range of sensitivities and specificities have been reported (for systematic review see Muayqil and colleagues[22]). Indeed, a highly elevated t-tau showed improved diagnostic accuracy for CJD compared with 14-3-3 in some studies.[23,24] This may be caused in part by differences in study populations (ie, use of autopsy confirmation for diagnostic accuracy) or other patient factors. Indeed, certain disease states may influence the sensitivity of CSF 14-3-3 for CJD; CSF 14-3-3 accuracy is lower for younger patients, those with longer disease duration, and those with a specific genetic polymorphism (heterozygosity at codon 129 in the PrP gene) for sporadic CJD.[25] Furthermore, the sensitivity of these biomarkers may be greater in later stages of the illness, so a negative test may be followed by repeat testing a few weeks later.[25] Thus, CSF testing for CJD is more informative for cases with a high index of suspicion[22] and negative testing does not rule out CJD from the differential diagnosis. Finally, novel assays for total PrP, unfolded normal PrP (ie, normal "cellular" PrP conformation [PrP^C]), and misfolded pathogenic PrP (abnromal "scrapie associated" PrP conformation [PrP^{SC}]) in CSF have shown promising results for improved diagnostic accuracy.[26–32]

Metabolic Disorders

Inborn errors of metabolism can sometimes present in adulthood with a range of neuropsychiatric symptoms (for a review, see Gray and colleagues[33]). Most metabolic disorders can be detected by blood and urinalysis for amino acid and organic acid metabolites and/or specific enzymatic assays; however, elevated CSF and plasma metabolites pyruvate and lactate may suggest a mitochondrial disease,[2] many of which can manifest as an encephalopathy with focal neurologic symptoms.[34] CSF lactate can also be elevated in other CNS diseases, such as stroke, seizures, and infection.

In summary, a detailed clinical history and examination, together with neuroimaging and other ancillary testing as appropriate, are critical to help narrow the differential diagnosis for specific RPD etiologies to direct further testing in CSF and help confirm diagnosis.

CEREBRAL BIOPSY FOR RAPIDLY PROGRESSIVE DEMENTIAS

If the clinical, radiologic, and body fluid testing have not resulted in a specific diagnosis, and diagnosis is vital to choosing an outcome-influencing treatment (eg, immunosuppression for an autoimmune cause vs antibacterial/fungal treatments for an infectious cause), a brain biopsy may be considered. Before choosing biopsy, it must be noted that only about 60% to 80% of biopsies result in a specific diagnosis,[35,36] and that 11% to 21% of biopsies are associated with transient postbiopsy complications, such as wound infection and seizure,[35] although others report lower rates of complications when skilled surgeons performed the procedure.[3] Furthermore, in case of suspicion of CJD, safety of the health personnel and cost of disposal of instruments are also factors to take into consideration.

Among the vascular conditions, biopsy may be used to establish diagnosis of cerebral amyloid angiopathy and cerebral vasculitis.[1,6] For primary CNS vasculitis, diagnosis is often by angiography, although biopsy (including the dura, leptomeninges, cortex, and white matter) may be used for confirmation[7]; and diagnostic sensitivity is improved when radiographically abnormal areas are targeted for biopsy.[3] In infectious cases where CSF and serum analyses fail to detect the organism, PCR on a biopsy sample may be useful.[37,38] In sarcoidosis and brain neoplasias (including PCNSL, intravascular lymphoma, and gliomatosis cerebri), brain biopsy may be needed for definite diagnosis.[1,6] For example, a low-grade T-cell lymphoma with unremarkable cytomorphology may not be recognized on a small biopsy unless T-cell receptor gene rearrangements are tested for.[35] In prion disease, definitive diagnosis is by demonstration of prion protein (PrP^{sc}) aggregations with spongiosis in the brain. PrP^{sc} can also be detected in tonsillar tissue for vCJD.[6] Other nonbrain biopsies useful for diagnosis include jejunal biopsy for Whipple disease, small bowel biopsy for gluten sensitivity dementia, and lip biopsy for Sjögren encephalopathy.[7]

CEREBROSPINAL FLUID BIOMARKERS FOR NEURODEGENERATIVE DISEASE

A key characteristic of neurodegenerative diseases is the accumulation and aggregation of naturally occurring proteins within the CNS. Indeed, modern immunohistochemical stains use antibodies directed at these key proteins (ie, tau, α-synuclein, amyloid-β, TDP-43) for neuropathologic diagnosis.[39] Furthermore, recent animal and cell model experiments have found evidence to suggest that the neuron-to-neuron spread of these proteins within the CNS may be a central feature of disease pathogenesis.[40,41] These in vivo/in vitro studies compliment neuropathologic staging systems proposed for AD, PD, FTD, and ALS, where there is evidence of a nonrandom hierarchical deposition of neurodegenerative disease protein aggregates within the CNS that correlate with clinical symptoms and disease progression.[42–45] Despite the similarity of transmission between neurons of neurodegenerative disease and prion disease, there is currently no evidence of transmission of clinical AD, PD, FTD, or ALS between humans or nonhuman primates.[46] As we move toward development of disease-modifying therapies that target the pathologic aggregation of specific neurodegenerative proteins, antemortem diagnosis is critical. CSF analysis provides a relatively noninvasive method to potentially measure these proteins, which could aid in diagnosis.

The most extensive experience with CSF biomarkers in neurodegenerative disease is with measurement of the AD-associated proteins, tau and amyloid-β (Aβ_{1-42}). Several large-scale studies have found evidence that AD is associated with increased levels of tau and decreased levels of Aβ_{1-42}.[47–49] Tau exists in six different isoforms and has several amino acid residues that can be modified by phosphorylation (for review see Yoshiyama and coworkers[50]). T-tau is measured using capture antibodies specific for regions found in all six isoforms (ie, proline 218–lysine 224) and not specific for phosphorylation modifications, presumably measuring all forms of tau in CSF. Although Phosphorylated-tau (p-tau) is measured using capture antibodies specific for phosphorylation epitopes (ie, threonine 181 or threonine 231), t-tau elevation may be a more general marker for neurodegeneration and injury because elevations are seen following head injury, stroke, infections, AD, and prion disease.[51–53] Tau is highly phosphorylated in AD brain tissue[54] and thus, p-tau may be a more specific marker for AD neuropathology. There seems to be a direct correlation of CSF t-tau/ p-tau and inverse correlation of CSF Aβ_{1-42} levels with the severity of neurofibrillary tau and amyloid plaque pathology in the brain, as evidenced by biopsy samples in patients evaluated for normal pressure hydrocephalus[55] and in vivo amyloid imaging.[56] Therefore, it is hypothesized that t-tau/p-tau levels are associated with release of these proteins from degenerating neurons, whereas Aβ_{1-42} is sequestered in extracellular plaques resulting in lower CSF levels.

Large-scale studies have found evidence that higher t-tau to $A\beta_{1-42}$ or p-tau to $A\beta_{1-42}$ ratios in CSF have high sensitivity and specificity to differentiate AD from healthy control subjects.[47] Furthermore, in patients with mild cognitive impairments this CSF biomarker profile may be useful in predicting risk of conversion to AD.[49] Thus, CSF analysis may be useful to identify patients with preclinical disease.[57] Despite this growing body of data on the potential clinical use of these CSF markers the official recommendations from the Alzheimer's Association and National Institutes of Health National Institute on Aging reserve the use of CSF t-tau, p-tau, and $A\beta_{1-42}$ analysis for research purposes only.[57,58] There are several reasons for this determination. Currently, these analytes can be measured by several different immunoassay platforms. Absolute levels of CSF t-tau, p-tau, and $A\beta_{1-42}$ differ between platforms, but are highly correlated and may be transformed into equivalent units.[59] Research data show an acceptable range of variance in these assays within most laboratories but there are many potential sources of within- and between-laboratory error at pre-analytical, analytical, and postanalytical steps that require correction before these tests can be put to clinical use. Indeed, there have been US and international efforts to develop uniform measures of CSF collection and analyses between laboratories.[60–62] Development and implementation of standard operating procedures for CSF collection have been very successful in the Alzheimer's Disease Neuroimaging Initiative studies.[48] Future efforts such as these will likely provide a standardized analytical approach that will be acceptable for clinical use.

Another potential limitation of CSF biomarkers in neurodegenerative disease is the minimal knowledge of longitudinal change of the analytes during the course of disease. Despite evidence for CSF abnormalities in preclinical disease, few studies have examined longitudinal change in CSF t-tau, p-tau, and $A\beta_{1-42}$ in AD[63–65] but suggest these analytes may be relatively static during the symptomatic phase of the disease for most patients. As such, longitudinal studies of AD,[48] PD,[66] and those currently in development for FTD will be instrumental in furthering the understanding of CSF biomarker levels throughout the course of disease.

There is considerable clinical overlap between AD and FTD making the clinical differentiation of these conditions difficult. Several studies have found that an elevated t-tau to $A\beta_{1-42}$ ratio can also help differentiate neuropathologically confirmed cases of AD from FTD.[59,67,68] FTD clinical syndromes are caused by two major classes of proteinopathy: those with pathologic inclusions composed of tau (FTLD-Tau) or TDP-43 (FTLD-TDP),[69] which cannot be readily differentiated during life. FTLD-Tau has similar hyperphosphorylation of tau to AD; however, CSF p-tau levels are not typically as high as in AD.[68] Direct comparison of FTLD-Tau and FTLD-TDP autopsy cases finds diagnostic use of the ratio of p-tau to t-tau, with FTLD-TDP having lower p-tau levels presumably because these cases lack abnormal hyperphosphorylation of tau.[70] In addition, ALS is also characterized by TDP-43 pathology in the spinal cord and motor cortex and also has lower p-tau in the CSF compared with FTLD-Tau and healthy control subjects.[71] These studies suggest AD-associated CSF analytes may have clinical use in ALS/FTD but there is still a need for FTD-ALS–specific biomarkers. Indeed, comorbid AD neuropathology is not uncommon among cases of FTD-ALS and may influence CSF analyte levels.[67] Efforts to detect TDP-43 in the CSF have not been effective in differentiating FTD-ALS from control subjects,[72] but perhaps future efforts directed at disease-specific epitopes for TDP-43 will be clinically useful, because detection of specific forms and modifications of the tau protein that are unique to FTLD-Tau show preliminary evidence for diagnostic utility.[73,74] Future work using CSF samples from autopsy-confirmed cases of FTD-ALS will be critical for the development of FTD-ALS specific biomarkers.

CSF analytes of t-tau, p-tau, and $A\beta_{1-42}$ may have clinical use in synucleinopathies (ie, PD, DLB). There is considerable clinical and pathologic overlap between PD, DLB, and AD, with a large number of cases having significant amounts of AD-associated plaque and tangle pathology, which may influence cognitive symptoms and development of dementia (PD dementia).[75] Indeed, PD dementia was found to be associated with higher CSF t-tau and p-tau, and lower CSF $A\beta_{1-42}$ than PD cases.[76,77] The levels of these analytes seem to be intermediate to those in patients with AD and healthy control subjects.[76,77] An AD-associated CSF profile (ie, increased t-tau to $A\beta_{1-42}$ ratio) was found in a higher percentage of PD dementia cases than PD cases[78] and a prospective study found that low CSF $A\beta_{1-42}$ levels that indicate AD predict cognitive decline in PD across several cognitive domains.[79] Thus, the levels of CSF tau and $A\beta_{1-42}$ that are associated with AD may have predictive value for cognitive decline in PD.

Immunoassays have been developed to detect forms of the protein α-synuclein, which is found in the characteristic Lewy body inclusions in PD/PD dementia/DLB.[80] CSF levels of αsynuclein are generally lower in PD/PD dementia/DLB compared with control subjects[76,81] but there seems to be considerable overlap, which may limit diagnostic use; however, it may be useful in differentiating DLB and AD.[76,82] Interestingly, drug-naive patients with early stage PD without dementia also have lower levels of CSF t-tau than control subjects, and these low levels of tau correlate with lower CSF levels of αsynuclein,[81] thus reinforcing the clinicopathologic overlap of AD and PD-DLB. Oligomeric or aggregations of multiple α-synuclein proteins have been measured in CSF and preliminarily seem to have some usefulness in diagnosis of PD.[83] Future studies in large autopsy-confirmed cohorts are required to help clarify and confirm these results.

Finally, exploratory approaches using multiplexed assays to simultaneously measure numerous analytes related to neurodegeneration, such as cytokines and neuropeptides, have found several potential novel CSF analytes that may be useful in the diagnosis of neurodegenerative diseases.[84,85] These types of approaches do not have an a priori hypothesis for analyte selection and are useful to discover potential novel analytes but require further validation in large-scale studies. Because the gold standard for all neurodegenerative diseases is autopsy, CSF samples from autopsy-confirmed cases of neurodegenerative disease are an extremely valuable resource for research. Any potential CSF biomarker for these conditions requires thorough validation in several large independent patient cohorts and standardization of CSF collection and assay parameters to ensure clinical reliability between laboratories.

SUMMARY

CSF analysis is an important tool, not only in differentiating neurodegenerative disease from nondegenerative mimics (RPDs), but also is a potentially useful means for biomarker development for neurodegenerative conditions. A careful clinical evaluation is critical for all patients who present with cognitive and/or motor symptoms to help direct further diagnostics to exclude or confirm RPDs. Furthermore, CSF biomarker research has grown tremendously in recent years, and while currently reserved for research studies, future efforts will likely lead to novel clinical tests to improve the antemortem diagnosis of AD, PD, DLB, FTD, and ALS. This is critical for the implementation and evaluation of emerging disease-modifying therapies that target the abnormal aggregation and spread of neurodegenerative disease–associated proteins (ie, tau, amyloid-β, α-synuclein, and TDP-43).

REFERENCES

1. Paterson RW, Takada LT, Geschwind MD. Diagnosis and treatment of rapidly progressive dementias. Neurol Clin Pract 2012;2:187–200.
2. Rosenbloom MH, Atri A. The evaluation of rapidly progressive dementia. Neurologist 2011;17:67–74.
3. Salvarani C, Brown RD, Hunder GG. Adult primary central nervous system vasculitis. Lancet 2012;380:767–77.
4. Berlit P. Diagnosis and treatment of cerebral vasculitis. Ther Adv Neurol Disord 2010;3:29–42.
5. Tamagno G, Federspil G, Murialdo G. Clinical and diagnostic aspects of encephalopathy associated with autoimmune thyroid disease (or Hashimoto's encephalopathy). Intern Emerg Med 2006;1:15–23.
6. Geschwind MD, Shu H, Haman A, et al. Rapidly progressive dementia. Ann Neurol 2008;64:97–108.
7. Rosenbloom MH, Smith S, Akdal G, et al. Immunologically mediated dementias. Curr Neurol Neurosci Rep 2009;9:359–67.
8. West SG, Emlen W, Wener MH, et al. Neuropsychiatric lupus erythematosus: a 10-year prospective study on the value of diagnostic tests. Am J Med 1995;99: 153–63.
9. Zajicek JP, Scolding NJ, Foster O, et al. Central nervous system sarcoidosis: diagnosis and management. QJM 1999;92:103–17.
10. Tüzün E, Dalmau J. Limbic encephalitis and variants: classification, diagnosis and treatment. Neurologist 2007;13:261–71.
11. Thieben MJ, Lennon VA, Boeve BF, et al. Potentially reversible autoimmune limbic encephalitis with neuronal potassium channel antibody. Neurology 2004;62: 1177–82.
12. Dalmau J, Gleichman AJ, Hughes EG, et al. Anti-NMDA-receptor encephalitis: case series and analysis of the effects of antibodies. Lancet Neurol 2008;7: 1091–8.
13. Pelosof LC, Gerber DE. Paraneoplastic syndromes: an approach to diagnosis and treatment. Mayo Clin Proc 2010;85:838–54.
14. Rollins KE, Kleinschmidt-DeMasters BK, Corboy JR, et al. Lymphomatosis cerebri as a cause of white matter dementia. Hum Pathol 2005;36:282–90.
15. Antinori A, Arendt G, Becker JT, et al. Updated research nosology for HIV-associated neurocognitive disorders. Neurology 2007;69:1789–99.
16. Yao K, Honarmand S, Espinosa A, et al. Detection of human herpesvirus-6 in cerebrospinal fluid of patients with encephalitis. Ann Neurol 2009;65:257–67.
17. Berger JR, Aksamit AJ, Clifford DB, et al. PML diagnostic criteria: consensus statement from the AAN Neuroinfectious Disease Section. Neurology 2013;80: 1430–8.
18. Cho TA, Mckendall RR. Clinical approach to the syndromes of viral encephalitis, myelitis, and meningitis. Handb Clin Neurol 2014;123:89–121.
19. Benito-León J, Sedano LF, Louis ED. Isolated central nervous system Whipple's disease causing reversible frontotemporal-like dementia. Clin Neurol Neurosurg 2008;110:747–9.
20. Zerr I, Kallenberg K, Summers DM, et al. Updated clinical diagnostic criteria for sporadic Creutzfeldt-Jakob disease. Brain 2009;132:2659–68.
21. World Health Organization. WHO manual for surveillance of human transmissible spongiform encephalopathies including variant Creutzfeldt-Jakob disease. Geneva, Switzerland: World Health Organization; 2003.

22. Muayqil T, Gronseth G, Camicioli R. Evidence-based guideline: diagnostic accuracy of CSF 14-3-3 protein in sporadic Creutzfeldt-Jakob disease: report of the guideline development subcommittee of the American Academy of Neurology. Neurology 2012;79:1499–506.
23. Hamlin C, Puoti G, Berri S, et al. A comparison of tau and 14-3-3 protein in the diagnosis of Creutzfeldt-Jakob disease. Neurology 2012;79:547–52.
24. Skillbäck T, Rosén C, Asztely F, et al. Diagnostic performance of cerebrospinal fluid total tau and phosphorylated tau in Creutzfeldt-Jakob disease: results from the Swedish Mortality Registry. JAMA Neurol 2014;71:476–83.
25. Sanchez-Juan P, Green A, Ladogana A, et al. CSF tests in the differential diagnosis of Creutzfeldt-Jakob disease. Neurology 2006;67:637–43.
26. Llorens F, Ansoleaga B, Garcia-Esparcia P, et al. PrP mRNA and protein expression in brain and PrP(c) in CSF in Creutzfeldt-Jakob disease MM1 and VV2. Prion 2013;7:383–93.
27. Torres M, Cartier L, Matamala JM, et al. Altered Prion protein expression pattern in CSF as a biomarker for Creutzfeldt-Jakob disease. PLoS One 2012;7:e36159.
28. Meyne F, Gloeckner SF, Ciesielczyk B, et al. Total prion protein levels in the cerebrospinal fluid are reduced in patients with various neurological disorders. J Alzheimers Dis 2009;17:863–73.
29. Atarashi R, Satoh K, Sano K, et al. Ultrasensitive human prion detection in cerebrospinal fluid by real-time quaking-induced conversion. Nat Med 2011;17:175–8.
30. McGuire LI, Peden AH, Orrú CD, et al. Real time quaking-induced conversion analysis of cerebrospinal fluid in sporadic Creutzfeldt-Jakob disease. Ann Neurol 2012;72:278–85.
31. Sano K, Satoh K, Atarashi R, et al. Early detection of abnormal prion protein in genetic human prion diseases now possible using real-time QUIC assay. PLoS One 2013;8:e54915.
32. Dorey A, Tholance Y, Vighetto A, et al. Association of cerebrospinal fluid prion protein levels and the distinction between Alzheimer disease and Creutzfeldt-Jakob disease. JAMA Neurol 2015. http://dx.doi.org/10.1001/jamaneurol.2014.4068.
33. Gray RG, Preece MA, Green SH, et al. Inborn errors of metabolism as a cause of neurological disease in adults: an approach to investigation. J Neurol Neurosurg Psychiatry 2000;69:5–12.
34. Haas RH, Parikh S, Falk MJ, et al. Mitochondrial disease: a practical approach for primary care physicians. Pediatrics 2007;120:1326–33.
35. Schott JM, Reiniger L, Thom M, et al. Brain biopsy in dementia: clinical indications and diagnostic approach. Acta Neuropathol 2010;120:327–41.
36. Josephson SA, Papanastassiou AM, Berger MS, et al. The diagnostic utility of brain biopsy procedures in patients with rapidly deteriorating neurological conditions or dementia. J Neurosurg 2007;106:72–5.
37. Heckman GA, Hawkins C, Morris A, et al. Rapidly progressive dementia due to *Mycobacterium neoaurum* meningoencephalitis. Emerg Infect Dis 2004;10:924–7.
38. Valcour V, Haman A, Cornes S, et al. A case of enteroviral meningoencephalitis presenting as rapidly progressive dementia. Nat Clin Pract Neurol 2008;4:399–403.
39. Montine TJ, Phelps CH, Beach TG, et al. National Institute on Aging-Alzheimer's Association guidelines for the neuropathologic assessment of Alzheimer's disease: a practical approach. Acta Neuropathol 2012;123:1–11.

40. Jucker M, Walker LC. Self-propagation of pathogenic protein aggregates in neurodegenerative diseases. Nature 2013;501:45–51.
41. Guo JL, Lee VM. Cell-to-cell transmission of pathogenic proteins in neurodegenerative diseases. Nat Med 2014;20:130–8.
42. Braak H, Braak E. Neuropathological stageing of Alzheimer-related changes. Acta Neuropathol 1991;82:239–59.
43. Braak H, Del Tredici K, Rüb U, et al. Staging of brain pathology related to sporadic Parkinson's disease. Neurobiol Aging 2003;24:197–211.
44. Brettschneider J, Del Tredici K, Irwin DJ, et al. Sequential distribution of pTDP-43 pathology in behavioral variant frontotemporal dementia (bvFTD). Acta Neuropathol 2014;127:423–39.
45. Brettschneider J, Del Tredici K, Toledo JB, et al. Stages of pTDP-43 pathology in amyotrophic lateral sclerosis. Ann Neurol 2013;74:20–38.
46. Irwin DJ, Abrams JY, Schonberger LB, et al. Evaluation of potential infectivity of Alzheimer and Parkinson disease proteins in recipients of cadaver-derived human growth hormone. JAMA Neurol 2013;70:462–8.
47. Shaw LM, Vanderstichele H, Knapik-Czajka M, et al. Cerebrospinal fluid biomarker signature in Alzheimer's disease neuroimaging initiative subjects. Ann Neurol 2009;65:403–13.
48. Trojanowski JQ, Vandeerstichele H, Korecka M, et al. Update on the biomarker core of the Alzheimer's Disease Neuroimaging Initiative subjects. Alzheimers Dement 2010;6:230–8.
49. De Meyer G, Shapiro F, Vanderstichele H, et al. Diagnosis-independent Alzheimer disease biomarker signature in cognitively normal elderly people. Arch Neurol 2010;67:949–56.
50. Yoshiyama Y, Lee VM, Trojanowski JQ. Therapeutic strategies for tau mediated neurodegeneration. J Neurol Neurosurg Psychiatr 2013;84:784–95.
51. Hesse C, Rosengren L, Vanmechelen E, et al. Cerebrospinal fluid markers for Alzheimer's disease evaluated after acute ischemic stroke. J Alzheimers Dis 2000;2: 199–206.
52. Ost M, Nylén K, Csajbok L, et al. Initial CSF total tau correlates with 1-year outcome in patients with traumatic brain injury. Neurology 2006;67:1600–4.
53. Krut JJ, Zetterberg H, Blennow K, et al. Cerebrospinal fluid Alzheimer's biomarker profiles in CNS infections. J Neurol 2013;260:620–6.
54. Matsuo ES, Shin RW, Billingsley ML, et al. Biopsy-derived adult human brain tau is phosphorylated at many of the same sites as Alzheimer's disease paired helical filament tau. Neuron 1994;13:989–1002.
55. Hamilton R, Patel S, Lee EB, et al. Lack of shunt response in suspected idiopathic normal pressure hydrocephalus with Alzheimer disease pathology. Ann Neurol 2010;68:535–40.
56. Fagan AM, Mintun MA, Mach RH, et al. Inverse relation between in vivo amyloid imaging load and cerebrospinal fluid Abeta42 in humans. Ann Neurol 2006;59: 512–9.
57. Sperling RA, Aisen PS, Beckett LA, et al. Toward defining the preclinical stages of Alzheimer's disease: recommendations from the National Institute on Aging-Alzheimer's Association workgroups on diagnostic guidelines for Alzheimer's disease. Alzheimers Dement 2011;7:280–92.
58. McKhann GM, Knopman DS, Chertkow H, et al. The diagnosis of dementia due to Alzheimer's disease: recommendations from the National Institute on Aging-Alzheimer's Association workgroups on diagnostic guidelines for Alzheimer's disease. Alzheimers Dement 2011;7:263–9.

59. Irwin DJ, McMillan CT, Toledo JB, et al. Comparison of cerebrospinal fluid levels of tau and Aβ 1-42 in Alzheimer disease and frontotemporal degeneration using 2 analytical platforms. Arch Neurol 2012;69:1018–25.
60. Mattsson N, Andreasson U, Persson S, et al. The Alzheimer's Association external quality control program for cerebrospinal fluid biomarkers. Alzheimers Dement 2011;7:386–95.e6.
61. Shaw LM, Vanderstichele H, Knapik-Czajka M, et al. Qualification of the analytical and clinical performance of CSF biomarker analyses in ADNI. Acta Neuropathol 2011;121:597–609.
62. Vanderstichele H, Bibl M, Engelborghs S, et al. Standardization of preanalytical aspects of cerebrospinal fluid biomarker testing for Alzheimer's disease diagnosis: a consensus paper from the Alzheimer's Biomarkers Standardization Initiative. Alzheimers Dement 2012;8:65–73.
63. Le Bastard N, Aerts L, Sleegers K, et al. Longitudinal stability of cerebrospinal fluid biomarker levels: fulfilled requirement for pharmacodynamic markers in Alzheimer's disease. J Alzheimers Dis 2013;33:807–22.
64. Mattsson N, Portelius E, Rolstad S, et al. Longitudinal cerebrospinal fluid biomarkers over four years in mild cognitive impairment. J Alzheimers Dis 2012; 30:767–78.
65. Toledo JB, Xie SX, Trojanowski JQ, et al. Longitudinal change in CSF Tau and Aβ biomarkers for up to 48 months in ADNI. Acta Neuropathol 2013;126:659–70.
66. Parkinson Progression Marker Initiative. The Parkinson Progression Marker Initiative (PPMI). Prog Neurobiol 2011;95:629–35.
67. Toledo JB, Brettschneider J, Grossman M, et al. CSF biomarkers cutoffs: the importance of coincident neuropathological diseases. Acta Neuropathol 2012; 124:23–35.
68. Bian H, Van Swieten JC, Leight S, et al. CSF biomarkers in frontotemporal lobar degeneration with known pathology. Neurology 2008;70:1827–35.
69. Mackenzie IR, Neumann M, Bigio EH, et al. Nomenclature and nosology for neuropathologic subtypes of frontotemporal lobar degeneration: an update. Acta Neuropathol 2010;119:1–4.
70. Hu WT, Watts K, Grossman M, et al. Reduced CSF p-Tau181 to Tau ratio is a biomarker for FTLD-TDP. Neurology 2013;81:1945–52.
71. Grossman M, Elman L, McCluskey L, et al. Phosphorylated tau as a candidate biomarker for amyotrophic lateral sclerosis. JAMA Neurol 2014;71:442–8.
72. Steinacker P, Hendrich C, Sperfeld AD, et al. TDP-43 in cerebrospinal fluid of patients with frontotemporal lobar degeneration and amyotrophic lateral sclerosis. Arch Neurol 2008;65:1481–7.
73. Luk C, Compta Y, Magdalinou N, et al. Development and assessment of sensitive immuno-PCR assays for the quantification of cerebrospinal fluid three- and four-repeat tau isoforms in tauopathies. J Neurochem 2012;123:396–405.
74. Borroni B, Gardoni F, Parnetti L, et al. Pattern of Tau forms in CSF is altered in progressive supranuclear palsy. Neurobiol Aging 2009;30:34–40.
75. Irwin DJ, Lee VM, Trojanowski JQ. Parkinson's disease dementia: convergence of α-synuclein, tau and amyloid-β pathologies. Nat Rev Neurosci 2013;14:626–36.
76. Hall S, Öhrfelt A, Constantinescu R, et al. Accuracy of a panel of 5 cerebrospinal fluid biomarkers in the differential diagnosis of patients with dementia and/or parkinsonian disorders. Arch Neurol 2012;69:1445–52.
77. Compta Y, Martí MJ, Ibarretxe-Bilbao N, et al. Cerebrospinal tau, phospho-tau, and beta-amyloid and neuropsychological functions in Parkinson's disease. Mov Disord 2009;24:2203–10.

78. Montine TJ, Shi M, Quinn JF, et al. CSF Aβ(42) and tau in Parkinson's disease with cognitive impairment. Mov Disord 2010;25:2682–5.
79. Siderowf A, Xie SX, Hurtig H, et al. CSF amyloid {beta} 1-42 predicts cognitive decline in Parkinson disease. Neurology 2010;75:1055–61.
80. Mollenhauer B, Cullen V, Kahn I, et al. Direct quantification of CSF alpha-synuclein by ELISA and first cross-sectional study in patients with neurodegeneration. Exp Neurol 2008;213:315–25.
81. Kang JH, Irwin DJ, Chen-Plotkin AS, et al. Association of cerebrospinal fluid β-amyloid 1-42, T-tau, P-tau181, and α-synuclein levels with clinical features of drug-naive patients with early Parkinson disease. JAMA Neurol 2013;70:1277–87.
82. Toledo JB, Korff A, Shaw LM, et al. CSF α-synuclein improves diagnostic and prognostic performance of CSF tau and Aβ in Alzheimer's disease. Acta Neuropathol 2013;126:683–97.
83. Tokuda T, Qureshi MM, Ardah MT, et al. Detection of elevated levels of α-synuclein oligomers in CSF from patients with Parkinson disease. Neurology 2010;75:1766–72.
84. Hu WT, Chen-Plotkin A, Grossman M, et al. Novel CSF biomarkers for frontotemporal lobar degenerations. Neurology 2010;75:2079–86.
85. Hu WT, Chen-Plotkin A, Arnold SE, et al. Novel CSF biomarkers for Alzheimer's disease and mild cognitive impairment. Acta Neuropathol 2010;119:669–78.

Neuropsychiatric Management of Young-Onset Dementias

Shunichiro Shinagawa, MD, PhD

KEYWORDS

- Young-onset dementia • Alzheimer's disease • Frontotemporal dementia
- Neuropsychiatric symptoms • Pharmacologic intervention
- Nonpharmacologic intervention

KEY POINTS

- Neuropsychiatric symptoms in patients with young-onset dementia (YOD) lead to a deterioration in everyday functions, affecting the patient and causing significant caregiver burden.
- Neuropsychiatric management of YOD patients should include pharmacologic and nonpharmacologic strategies.
- Nonpharmacologic interventions, including psychological management, environmental strategies, and caregiver's support, should be the first choice for neuropsychiatric management.
- Pharmacologic interventions, including cholinesterase inhibitors, N-methyl-D-aspartate antagonist, and other psychotropic drugs can treat cognitive and neuropsychiatric symptoms.
- Antipsychotics should be used carefully, particularly in patients who have dementia with Lewy bodies and frontotemporal dementia, because these forms are exquisitely sensitive to these drugs.

INTRODUCTION

Young-onset dementia (YOD) refers to patients diagnosed with dementia before 65 years of age. YOD is a relatively common, but frequently misdiagnosed, condition. Patients with YOD have more varied differential diagnoses than late-onset dementia, including not only Alzheimer disease (AD) but also frontotemporal dementia (FTD) syndrome, vascular dementia (VaD), dementia with Lewy bodies (DLB) or Parkinson disease dementia (PDD), traumatic head injury, alcohol-related dementia, and other

Conflict of Interest: The author has no conflict of interest to declare.
Department of Psychiatry, The Jikei University School of Medicine, 3-25-8 Nishi-shinbashi, Minato-ku, Tokyo 105-8461, Japan
E-mail address: shinagawa@jikei.ac.jp

Psychiatr Clin N Am 38 (2015) 323–331
http://dx.doi.org/10.1016/j.psc.2015.01.004
0193-953X/15/$ – see front matter © 2015 Elsevier Inc. All rights reserved.

conditions. Because patients with YOD often presents with neuropsychiatric features, including behavioral changes and psychiatric manifestations that sometimes precede and progress to cognitive decline, accurate diagnoses are difficult. These neuropsychiatric symptoms lead to deterioration of everyday functions, which affects not only the patient but also causes significant caregiver burden.

Thus, it is important to diagnose YOD accurately, particularly because different diagnoses result in different management and treatment options. Accurate differential diagnosis of YOD based on current symptoms, present history, past medical history, family history, neurologic examinations, cognitive tests, neuroimaging (such as brain CT or MRI), and laboratory investigations form the basis for neuropsychiatric management. It is particularly important to identify any treatable causes of dementia in the differential diagnosis, such as reactions to medications, metabolic abnormalities, nutritional deficiencies, infections, and normal pressure hydrocephalus.

Management of YOD can require pharmacologic and nonpharmacologic strategies. Pharmacologic interventions may work to reduce the impact or slow the progression of the disease. Pharmacologic interventions may also be needed to manage neuropsychiatric symptoms, sometimes called behavioral and psychological symptoms of dementia, such as delusions, hallucinations, agitation, and depression.

Nonpharmacologic management strategies include environmental strategies, which may be employed to minimize the consequences of neuropsychiatric symptoms; behavioral management and other interventions; caregiver's support; and community health services and institutional care. Long-term support is vital to help manage the cognitive and neuropsychiatric symptoms of YOD. A combination of pharmacologic treatments and nonpharmacologic approaches is necessary for the appropriate management of patients with YOD.

PHARMACOLOGIC INTERVENTIONS

Strategies for pharmacologic management of YOD are similar to those for late-onset dementia; currently, no YOD-specific pharmacologic therapies are available. In general, pharmacologic management strategies include the use of cholinesterase inhibitors (ChEls) and the N-methyl-D-aspartate (NMDA) antagonist, memantine (ie, antidementia drugs), and other psychotropic drugs to treat the neuropsychiatric symptoms. Pharmacologic interventions differ according to the underlying causes of dementia; these underlying causes should be treated appropriately. In addition, vascular risk factors can modify the progression of dementia, and thus it is important to pay close attention to these markers. It is also important to treat any comorbid medical condition or illness. Current antidementia agents for neurodegenerative diseases, such as AD or DLB/PDD, do not prevent or reverse these diseases; that is, they are not disease-modifying drugs. However, these drugs may offer symptomatic benefits for cognitive, global, functional, and neuropsychiatric outcome measures.

Antidementia Drugs for Alzheimer Disease

During the last decade, a large body of evidence has supported the use of antidementia medication in patients with AD (the most common cause of dementia). The current pharmacologic approach to AD treatment is based on symptomatic therapy using ChEls, such as donepezil, rivastigmine, galantamine, and memantine. Regardless of the pharmacotherapy, it is important to prescribe medications according to current guidelines and ensure routine follow-ups.

ChEls have proven to be the most worthwhile therapeutic agents for symptomatic improvements in AD because cholinergic deficits are a consistent and early finding in AD.[1] Clinical trials have shown significant improvements in cognitive, global, functional, and behavioral outcome measures after treatment with ChEls and memantine.[2] The available evidence shows that ChEls are effective across the spectrum of AD (mild, moderate, and severe) and several randomized, controlled studies have described modest, but significant, improvements in neuropsychiatric symptoms such as apathy, anxiety, and depression.[3] ChEls should be prescribed with caution in patients with sick sinus syndrome or other supraventricular conduction abnormalities, those who are susceptible to peptic ulcers, and those with asthma or chronic obstructive pulmonary disease.

Memantine, an NMDA receptor antagonist, may reduce glutamate-mediated neuronal excitotoxicity and result in modest symptomatic benefits for patients with moderate to severe AD.[4] Memantine is not indicated in patients with mild AD. Meta-analyses indicate that memantine may confer benefits in the treatment of mild to moderate irritability and mood swings, agitation or aggression, and psychosis in patients with AD.[5] This evidence is very encouraging, and suggests that memantine is a useful agent for the treatment for neuropsychiatric symptoms without the use of antipsychotics.[6]

Antipsychotics and Antidepressants

Although ChEls and memantine have some effect on neuropsychiatric symptoms, management of some neuropsychiatric symptoms in patients with dementia, such as agitation and psychosis, remain a challenge.

Antipsychotics

Antipsychotics or neuroleptics may be required if a patient exhibits refractory psychotic symptoms, poses a threat to themselves or others, or if other treatments, including nonpharmacologic management and other pharmacologic interventions, are not effective. Antipsychotics have been prescribed widely to treat neuropsychiatric symptoms; they were perceived to have potential benefits owing to their efficacy in treating psychosis in people with schizophrenia and bipolar disorder, and their sedative properties. Although the use of typical antipsychotics has declined, atypical antipsychotic drugs are frequently used in the pharmacologic treatment of neuropsychiatric symptoms. However, increasing safety concerns regarding use of this class of compounds in people with dementia has resulted in warnings from regulatory authorities. In 2005, the US Food and Drug Administration issued a warning regarding the increased risk of mortality associated with atypical antipsychotic use in patients with dementia; this warning was extended in 2008 to include typical antipsychotics. A large-scale, randomized, controlled trial concluded that adverse effects such as extrapyramidal signs, sedation, mental status change offset the advantages of antipsychotic use for the treatment of psychosis, aggression, or agitation in patients with AD.[7,8] Also, data from long-term, placebo-controlled trials found that patients with AD who are prescribed antipsychotic medication had an increased risk of mortality.[9]

On the basis of these safety concerns, we need to review clinical practice in this area. Antipsychotics should be used for the shortest time possible, at the lowest possible dose. Notably, patients with DLB (or PDD) and FTD are exquisitely sensitive to neuroleptics and can develop life-threatening extrapyramidal syndromes after use.

Antidepressants

Depression frequently accompanies all forms of YOD. Mood symptoms should be assessed specifically during consultations, and there should be a low threshold for treatment with antidepressants. The efficacy of antidepressants in treating depression in patients with dementia is not yet proven, because the evidence is inconclusive.[10–12] The accumulation of evidence suggests nonpharmacologic approaches may be effective for patients presenting with both mild to moderate depression and dementia. In cases of severe depression, or depression not managed through nonpharmacologic approaches, a trial of an antidepressant may be initiated.[13] Selective serotonin reuptake inhibitors are often used as a first-line pharmacologic treatment because of their favorable side effect profile and because antidepressants with strong anticholinergic effects may worsen cognition. Antidepressants may also be used to treat agitation and psychosis in people with dementia. Antidepressants seem to be well-tolerated compared with antipsychotics.[14]

Pharmacologic Interventions for Other Forms of Young-onset Dementia

Options for pharmacologic interventions to treat neuropsychiatric symptoms differ largely according to the causes of dementia; the underlying neuroanatomic and neurotransmitter mechanisms mediating these symptoms differ between diseases.

Frontotemporal dementia

FTD is a neurodegenerative disorder caused by focal degeneration of the frontal and anterior temporal lobes, and characterized by progressive changes in behavior, emotion, and personality, including early behavioral disinhibition, apathy, and loss of sympathy or empathy, as well as impulsive stereotypic behaviors and dietary changes.[15] Management of FTD is important because it is a common cause of YOD and has a similar incidence and prevalence to AD in the YOD cohort.[16]

To date, there is no specific treatment for FTD. Thus, medications typically prescribed for other types of dementia and psychiatric syndromes are used frequently as off-label treatments for FTD.[17] Current pharmacologic strategies for FTD have focused on modulation of the behavioral symptoms described. These medications include medication for AD, such as ChEIs and memantine, as well as antidepressants such as selective serotonin reuptake inhibitors, and atypical antipsychotics. However, the effects of these medications are variable and usually insufficient for treating the symptom profile. In general, antipsychotic use is often associated with adverse effect profiles. Specifically, there is an increased susceptibility to extrapyramidal symptoms after antipsychotic use in patients with FTD.[18] There is also the possibility that ChEIs may worsen behavioral disturbances in FTD.[19] Trials of memantine in FTD patients have not yet demonstrated clear benefits.[20,21] To date, implementation of drug trials has been challenging and most reports of FTD treatments are based on small case series; few large, double-blind, randomized, controlled trials have been conducted.

Dementia with Lewy bodies and Parkinson disease dementia

DLB is a common cause of dementia. The core clinical features of DLB include neuropsychiatric symptoms, such as visual hallucination and depression and motor symptoms of parkinsonism, as well as cognitive impairments characterized by deficits of attention, executive function, and visual perception.[22] Among these symptoms, fluctuating cognitive abilities, hallucinations, delusions, and depression are major sources of difficulties and distress for both patients and caregivers. The motor and autonomic features negatively affect daily activities, leading to poorer quality of life. However, pharmacologic management of DLB remains challenging because of the risk of adverse reactions to medication. Treatments for 1 aspect of the disease may exacerbate other symptoms.

It is well-recognized that DLB patients can be exquisitely sensitive to antipsychotics and can develop life-threatening sensitivities. On the other hand, antiparkinson medication prescribed to improve motor symptoms can exacerbate neuropsychiatric symptoms, such as visual hallucinations.

There are several randomized, controlled trials that report improvements in behavioral and cognitive symptoms in DLB after ChEI treatment.[23,24] Importantly, ChEIs can improve neuropsychiatric symptoms, such as visual hallucinations and delusions, in DLB patients. Thereby, donepezil, one of the ChEI agents, has been approved recently for treatment of DLB in Japan. To date, studies on memantine and DLB or PDD have been inconclusive.

Vascular dementia

VaD is a common cause of late-onset dementia and can also occur in YOD. Vascular risk factors, transient ischemic attacks, silent and clinically detected strokes, and ischemic changes are all associated with the development of dementia. Reports from clinical trials indicate that early treatment of hypertension, a risk factor for stroke, reduces VaD risk and slows progression.[25] However, unlike stroke, treatment of hyperlipidemia with statins or treatment of blood clotting abnormalities with acetylsalicylic acid do not seem to have an effect on VaD incidence or progression.[26] Currently, there are no pharmacologic agents with regulatory approval for treatment or prevention of VaD.

Pharmacologic agents for treatment of AD, such as ChEIs or memantine, may have, to some extent, positive effects on cognition in VaD. Cholinergic deficits in VaD are owing to ischemia of basal forebrain nuclei and cholinergic pathways and can be treated with ChEIs. Controlled clinical trials of ChEIs in patients with VaD, as well as in patients with AD and cardiovascular disease, have demonstrated improvements in cognition, behavior, and daily life activities.[27]

NONPHARMACOLOGIC INTERVENTIONS

Nonpharmacologic interventions may be equally as important as pharmacologic treatments in patients with YOD. An important aspect of nonpharmacologic management is acknowledgment of caregiver burden. Caregivers of YOD patients report a higher level of stress, burden, and depression compared with caregivers of people with late-onset dementia. This burden is likely owing to the high incidence of behavioral disturbances in YOD, combined with the fact that YOD strikes patients during their most productive years. Difficulties in caring for patients with YOD include the assumption that dementia is exclusively an illness of the elderly, high rates of misdiagnosis, lack of awareness from family members about how to deal with behavioral symptoms, increasing numbers of younger residents in nursing home and inadequate training of staff to care for them, insufficient funding for treatment programs, and limited advocacy in professional societies.[28] Psychological and emotional struggles, such as social isolation, are common as progressive disability and changes in behavior limit the patient and caregiver's interaction with others. Treatment of YOD must include caregivers, to ensure that they have access to community/home support and respite options.

Environmental Strategies

Environmental modifications play an important role in the management of YOD. Many studies have addressed the importance of environmental strategies, which may be used to minimize the effects of neuropsychiatric symptoms in patients with YOD.[29] It is difficult to conduct controlled studies of these environmental strategies because each patient faces a unique situation. As such, most of the descriptions herein are based on narrative and clinical experience and no controlled studies that assess the efficacy of these environmental strategies exist.

Safety

It is very important to assess safety in YOD, because patients often lack insight and demonstrate impaired judgment. First, clinicians and care staff should evaluate their behaviors in terms of threats to safety, as well as the frequency and duration of altered behaviors.[30] Physical safety around the home and in public should be considered. Most patients benefit from a stable and structured environment. For example, it is recommended that patients maintain a daily routine and that objects and furniture be kept in the same position. Disease stage should be taken into consideration when developing risk management strategies, because it may affect diverse aspects of a patient's daily life. In the earlier stages of YOD, decisions about safety and competence may be challenging. These decisions are best achieved with the assistance of a multidisciplinary team, including input from patients' families, nurses, speech therapists, and social workers.[31] Clinicians should be aware of the potential for self-harm, because YOD patients generally experience rapid disease progression and are likely to be confused about their situation. Despite its importance, there are no epidemiologic data about the prevalence of self-harm in patients with YOD, and further research is needed.

Finances

Different from patients with dementia in the elderly, patients with YOD tend to be working and have dependent children.[32] Therefore, YOD can bring unexpected reduction of income in their family and severe financial difficulty is common for their families. In addition to loss of income, financial issues may occur as a result of poor judgment, unnecessary spending, or forgetting bills, as well as the costs associated with providing care. Some patients with YOD face a serious dilemma before their diagnosis, as they lose their job owing to poor work performance, which in some countries results in the loss of health insurance. In this situation, it is important for medical professionals to ensure timely documentation of disability, to aid early retirement. Patients and families should consider their options for long-term care and other types of insurance.

Driving

In general, people with dementia gradually lose their capacity to drive a vehicle. However, this does not mean that a diagnosis of dementia should lead to an immediate recommendation to the patient to stop driving. They may still be capable of operating a vehicle at the time of diagnosis. Thus, the decision to stop driving should be made carefully, because it causes hardship by constraining patients' independence and life participation if done prematurely. It is important to examine each patient's driving capacity and driving behavior. Because patients may not have enough insight regarding their driving ability and may refuse to stop, it may worsen the relationship between patients and their families, as well as patient and their physicians.

Other Interventions

The benefit of increased physical activity has been demonstrated primarily for the prevention of AD and VaD, but less so for FTD.[9] However, given the growing body of evidence, exercise should be incorporated into a multifaceted treatment strategy for every YOD patient. Physical therapy may also help patients with mobility problems and reduce the risk of falls. There are many reports that some kind of nutrition and diet (such as the Mediterranean diet) may help to reduce the risk of developing AD and other causes of dementia.[33,34] However, there are currently no reports regarding diet or nutrition and YOD specifically.

Other therapies that have been shown to help alleviate neuropsychiatric symptoms in YOD patients include aromatherapy,[35] music therapy, recreation, bright light therapy, behavior therapy, reality orientation, reminiscence therapy, and art therapy.[36] A systematic review revealed that sensory interventions were effective in reducing agitation in AD, although this finding is not specific for patients with YOD.[37]

Services for People with Young-onset Disease

Home nursing or residential nursing care are often important resources for patients in the later stages of YOD, and their families. The ongoing support and care of people with YOD is complex and requires input from a multidisciplinary team. Patients and their families also benefit from support offered by voluntary organizations. However, there are few specific statutory services and a distinct lack of awareness and understanding about people who develop dementia at an early age, which makes it difficult for patients to access support. Younger people with dementia have different needs than older people with the disease. General dementia services are often inappropriate for use by younger people and may not meet their needs. Age can often be a barrier to accessing services, so younger people may not be eligible to receive care from general dementia services. Ideally, there would be widely available, regional specialist YOD services and flexible, "any age" services; some people over the age of 65 may be better served by services for younger people, whereas some people under the age of 65 may be better catered to by general dementia services.

SUMMARY

In the management of neuropsychiatric symptoms in YOD, nonpharmacologic interventions, including psychological management, environmental strategies, and caregiver support, should be the first choice of treatment. Pharmacologic agents should only be recommended when psychosocial interventions are inadequate. The type of dementia, individual symptom pattern, and drug tolerability should be considered when prescribing medication for people with YOD. Depending on the diagnostic syndrome and pathology to be treated, different types of drugs may improve different subsets of symptoms. Thus, there is an urgent need for more efficacious medications for the neuropsychiatric management of YOD.

REFERENCES

1. Whitehouse PJ, Price DL, Struble RG, et al. Alzheimers-disease and senile dementia - loss of neurons in the basal forebrain. Science 1982;215(4537):1237–9.
2. Birks J. Cholinesterase inhibitors for Alzheimer's disease. Cochrane Database Syst Rev 2006;(1):CD005593.
3. Rodda J, Morgan S, Walker Z. Are cholinesterase inhibitors effective in the management of the behavioral and psychological symptoms of dementia in

Alzheimer's disease? A systematic review of randomized, placebo-controlled trials of donepezil, rivastigmine and galantamine. Int Psychogeriatr 2009;21(5):813.

4. Kavirajan H. Memantine: a comprehensive review of safety and efficacy. Expert Opin Drug Saf 2009;8(1):89–109.

5. Gauthier S, Loft H, Cummings JL. Improvement in behavioural symptoms in patients with moderate to severe Alzheimer's disease by memantine: a pooled data analysis. Int J Geriatr Psychiatry 2008;23(5):537–45.

6. Corbett A, Smith J, Creese B, et al. Treatment of behavioral and psychological symptoms of Alzheimer's disease. Curr Treat Options Neurol 2012;14(2):113–25.

7. Schneider L, Tariot PN, Dagerman KS, et al. Effectiveness of atypical antipsychotic drugs in patients with Alzheimer's disease. N Engl J Med 2006;355(15):1525–38.

8. Ballard C, Hanney ML, Theodoulou M, et al. The dementia antipsychotic withdrawal trial (DART-AD): long-term follow-up of a randomised placebo-controlled trial. Lancet Neurol 2009;8(2):151–7.

9. Denkinger MD, Nikolaus T, Denkinger C, et al. Physical activity for the prevention of cognitive decline: current evidence from observational and controlled studies. Z Gerontol Geriatr 2011;45(1):11–6.

10. Banerjee S, Hellier J, Dewey M, et al. Sertraline or mirtazapine for depression in dementia (HTA-SADD): a randomised, multicentre, double-blind, placebo-controlled trial. Lancet 2011;378(9789):403–11.

11. Rosenberg PB, Drye LT, Martin BK, et al. Sertraline for the treatment of depression in Alzheimer disease. Am J Geriatr Psychiatry 2010;18(2):136–45.

12. Bains J, Birks J, Dening T. Antidepressants for treating depression in dementia. Cochrane Database Syst Rev 2008;(4):CD003944.

13. Leong C. Antidepressants for depression in patients with dementia: a review of the literature. Consult Pharm 2014;29(4):254–63.

14. Seitz DP, Adunuri N, Gill SS, et al. Antidepressants for agitation and psychosis in dementia. Cochrane Database Syst Rev 2011;(2):CD008191.

15. Shinagawa S. Phenotypic variety in the presentation of frontotemporal lobar degeneration. Int Rev Psychiatry 2013;25(2):138–44.

16. Ratnavalli E, Brayne C, Dawson K, et al. The prevalence of frontotemporal dementia. Neurology 2002;58(11):1615–21.

17. Hu B, Ross LL, Neuhaus J, et al. Off-label medication use in frontotemporal dementia. Am J Alzheimers Dis Other Demen 2010;25(2):128–33.

18. Kerssens CJ, Kerrsens CJ, Pijnenburg YA. Vulnerability to neuroleptic side effects in frontotemporal dementia. Eur J Neurol 2008;15(2):111–2.

19. Mendez MF, Shapira J, McMurtray A, et al. Preliminary findings: behavioral worsening on donepezil in patients with frontotemporal dementia. Am J Geriatr Psychiatry 2007;15(1):84–7.

20. Boxer AL, Knopman DS, Kaufer DI, et al. Memantine in patients with frontotemporal lobar degeneration: a multicentre, randomised, double-blind, placebo-controlled trial. Lancet Neurol 2013;12(2):149–56.

21. Vercelletto M, Boutoleau-Bretonnière C, Volteau C, et al. Memantine in behavioral variant frontotemporal dementia: negative results. J Alzheimers Dis 2011;23(4):749–59.

22. McKeith IG, Dickson DW, Lowe J, et al. Diagnosis and management of dementia with Lewy bodies: third report of the DLB consortium. Neurology 2005;65(12):1863–72.

23. McKeith I, del Ser T, Spano P, et al. Efficacy of rivastigmine in dementia with Lewy bodies: a randomised, double-blind, placebo-controlled international study. Lancet 2000;356(9247):2031–6.

24. Mori E, Ikeda M, Kosaka K, Donepezil-DLB Study Investigators. Donepezil for dementia with Lewy bodies: a randomized, placebo-controlled trial. Ann Neurol 2012;72(1):41–52.
25. Kirshner HS. Vascular dementia: a review of recent evidence for prevention and treatment. Curr Neurol Neurosci Rep 2009;9(6):437–42.
26. Baskys A, Cheng J-X. Pharmacological prevention and treatment of vascular dementia: approaches and perspectives. Exp Gerontol 2012;47(11):887–91.
27. Erkinjuntti TJ, Roman G, Gauthier S. Treatment of vascular dementia—evidence from clinical trials with cholinesterase inhibitors. J Neurol Sci 2003;226(1):63–6.
28. Chemali Z, Withall A, Daffner KR. The plight of caring for young patients with frontotemporal dementia. Am J Alzheimers Dis Other Demen 2010;25(2):109–15.
29. Ballard CG, Khan Z, Clack H, et al. Nonpharmacological treatment of Alzheimer disease. Can J Psychiatry 2011;56(10):589–95.
30. Talerico KA, Evans LK. Responding to safety issues in frontotemporal dementias. Neurology 2001;56(11):S52–5.
31. Henry M, Beeson PM, Rapcsak S. Treatment for Anomia in Semantic Dementia. Semin Speech Lang 2008;29(1):60–70.
32. Wylie MA, Shnall A, Onyike CU, et al. Management of frontotemporal dementia in mental health and multidisciplinary settings. Int Rev Psychiatry 2013;25(2):230–6.
33. Shah R. The role of nutrition and diet in Alzheimer disease: a systematic review. J Am Med Dir Assoc 2013;14(6):398–402.
34. Lourida I, Soni M, Thompson-Coon J, et al. Mediterranean Diet, cognitive function, and dementia. Epidemiology 2013;24(4):479–89.
35. Burns A, Perry E, Holmes C, et al. A double-blind placebo-controlled randomized trial of Melissa officinalis oil and donepezil for the treatment of agitation in Alzheimer's disease. Dement Geriatr Cogn Disord 2011;31(2):158–64.
36. Woods B. Invited commentary on: non-pharmacological interventions in dementia. Adv Psychiatr Treat 2004;10(3):178–9.
37. Kong EH, Evans LK, Guevara JP. Nonpharmacological intervention for agitation in dementia: a systematic review and meta-analysis. Aging Ment Health 2009;13(4):512–20.

The CARE Pathway Model for Dementia

Psychosocial and Rehabilitative Strategies for Care in Young-Onset Dementias

Darby Morhardt, PhD[a], Sandra Weintraub, PhD[a,b,c],
Becky Khayum, MS, CCC-SLP[d], Jaimie Robinson, MSW[e],
Jennifer Medina, PhD[a], Mary O'Hara, AM[a], Marsel Mesulam, MD[a,c],
Emily J. Rogalski, PhD[a,*]

KEYWORDS

- Quality of life • Neurocognitive profile • Symptom-specific strategies
- Clinical care model • Primary progressive aphasia
- Behavioral variant frontotemporal dementia • Posterior cortical atrophy
- Dementia of the Alzheimer type

KEY POINTS

- Individuals with young-onset dementia can differ dramatically in the types of symptoms they express; therefore, a one-size-fits-all model of care for dementia is inadequate for this population.
- The Care Pathway Model for Dementia (CARE-D) prescribes tailored care based on results from psychosocial and neuropsychological assessments.
- Interventions focus on a person's abilities and strengths and are adapted over time as needs and abilities change.
- The psychosocial context is an essential component. Consideration should be given to the living situation, social supports, life stage, financial resources, and individual's and family's preexisting coping strategies.
- The goal is to enhance quality of life by maximizing independence and safety, identifying helpful modifications to activities and the environment, and providing emotional support for individuals with young-onset dementia and their families.

Disclosures: B. Khayum is the president and a speech pathologist of MemoryCare Corporation. The other authors have no disclosures to report.
[a] Cognitive Neurology and Alzheimer's Disease Center, Northwestern University Feinberg School of Medicine, 320 East Superior Street, Searle Building 11th Floor, Chicago, IL 60611, USA; [b] Department of Psychiatry and Behavioral Sciences, Northwestern University Feinberg School of Medicine, 446 East Ontario, Chicago, IL 60611, USA; [c] Department of Neurology, Northwestern University Feinberg School of Medicine, 710 North Lake Shore Drive, Chicago, IL 60611, USA; [d] MemoryCare Corporation, 634 Brooklyn Drive, Aurora, IL 60502, USA; [e] Christ Hospital Cancer Center, 2139 Auburn Avenue, Cincinnati, OH 45219, USA
* Corresponding author.
E-mail address: erogalski@gmail.com

Psychiatr Clin N Am 38 (2015) 333–352
http://dx.doi.org/10.1016/j.psc.2015.01.005
psych.theclinics.com

Abbreviations	
bvFTD	Behavioral variant frontotemporal dementia
CARE-D	Care Pathway Model for Dementia
DAT	Dementia of the Alzheimer type
LBD	Cortical Lewy body disease
PCA	Posterior cortical atrophy
PPA	Primary progressive aphasia
WCST	Wisconsin Card Sorting Test

INTRODUCTION

Although aging is the leading risk factor for Alzheimer disease, it is estimated that at least 200,000 people under age 65 have what is commonly known as young-onset dementia.[1] Individuals with young-onset dementia can differ dramatically from those with older onset in the types of symptoms they express. Even those with the same clinical diagnosis (eg, dementia of the Alzheimer type [DAT]) can present with different neurocognitive profiles of impairment.[2–4] Individuals with young-onset dementia and their families have different needs, concerns, and access to resources than older adults who develop dementia.[5] This fact is related not only to the type of symptoms expressed but also to the time of life when the illness strikes. Individuals with young-onset dementia are likely to be healthier than individuals with late-onset dementia and less likely to have coexisting illnesses, such as cardiovascular disease, diabetes, or hearing loss and other sensory changes, making them good candidates for targeted therapies. Unfortunately, most psychosocial models of dementia care and intervention focus on a clinical diagnosis, usually dementia or Alzheimer disease dementia, without paying attention to the specific presenting symptoms. This approach may place individuals into programs or services solely based on a dementia diagnosis, regardless of whether or not a person is cognitively suited or age-appropriate for the intervention. One exception is the Tailored Activity Program.[6] This program trains occupational therapists to assess persons with dementia who exhibit behavioral symptoms for preserved capabilities that are then used to customize activities. The family and environment are included and considered critical to the intervention's success. Similarly, the CARE-D model identifies and builds on strengths based on a person's neurocognitive/behavioral profile and incorporates the family and environmental capacities; however, skills of both occupational therapists and speech-language pathologists are engaged to tailor appropriate interventions.

This article describes the conceptual design and implementation of CARE-D. The model is built on a framework provided by the neuropsychological characterization of cognitive and behavioral strengths and weaknesses in the early stages of illness and on a comprehensive psychosocial assessment (**Fig. 1**).

The model rests on the theory that psychosocial and rehabilitative interventions should address individual symptoms and distinctive neuropsychological profiles to improve quality of life and daily functioning for both the diagnosed individual and the family.[3,7,8] Although the model is targeted at mild and moderate stages of a dementia where there may be only one major area of difficulty, it can still be used in later stages when there are more cognitive and behavioral limitations and where the goal is to identify the most disruptive symptom needing intervention.

CARE-D was developed in a multidisciplinary outpatient clinical setting of behavioral neurologists, neuropsychologists, neuropsychiatrists, and social workers and

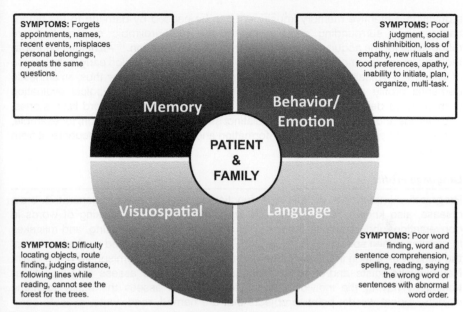

SYMPTOMS: Forgets appointments, names, recent events, misplaces personal belongings, repeats the same questions.

SYMPTOMS: Poor judgment, social dishinhibition, loss of empathy, new rituals and food preferences, apathy, inability to initiate, plan, organize, multi-task.

Memory

Behavior/ Emotion

PATIENT & FAMILY

Visuospatial

Language

SYMPTOMS: Difficulty locating objects, route finding, judging distance, following lines while reading, cannot see the forest for the trees.

SYMPTOMS: Poor word finding, word and sentence comprehension, spelling, reading, saying the wrong word or sentences with abnormal word order.

Fig. 1. The Care Pathway Model for Dementia (CARE-D).

relies on input from different members of the team. CARE-D has 3 components: (1) determination of a patient's neurocognitive profile; (2) psychosocial assessment; and (3) development of specific recommendations and strategies based on a patient's strengths and weaknesses within the context of the social network and environment.

Although any cognitive, behavioral, and motor symptoms can mark the earliest stages of a dementia, this article focus on 4 profiles that have well-established diagnostic criteria and good evidence of their symptoms, course, and biological features: progressive memory, language, visuospatial, and executive/behavioral/comportmental dysfunction. The clinical syndromes that embody these major domains of impairment are DAT, a memory dementia; primary progressive aphasia (PPA), a language dementia; posterior cortical atrophy (PCA), a visuospatial dementia; and behavioral variant frontotemporal dementia (bvFTD), a behavioral-social dementia.[3,9–14] Changes in mood, motor function, and sleep patterns also can be present in any of these profiles and need to be addressed in treatment planning but are discussed only briefly.

DETERMINATION OF A PATIENT'S NEUROCOGNITIVE PROFILE

The neurocognitive evaluation is completed by a neuropsychologist who conducts a detailed review of attention, language, memory, executive functions, visuospatial skills, and reasoning. A behavioral neurologist or neuropsychiatrist can often identify major areas of weakness with a briefer examination but may not include some of the process analysis that is derived from the neuropsychological evaluation. Findings from these examinations aid in identifying a patient's strengths and weaknesses so that the appropriate dementia care pathway can be implemented.

Memory Profile

Perhaps the most common early symptom of neurodegenerative dementia is amnesia, or loss of episodic, short-term (retentive) memory not due to inattentiveness or lack of motivation. Retentive memory impairment can be caused by damage to the hippocampus and surrounding components of the temporolimbic system that are responsible for the acquisition and retention of new information.[15] Alzheimer neuropathology, for reasons not well understood,[16] often targets this region early in the course of illness and typically starts by causing a progressive memory loss; thus, an amnestic dementia profile also is referred to as DAT. The neuropsychological evaluation demonstrates deficits on tests of learning and delayed recall of word lists, stories, and designs and differentiates among distinct stages of memory function, for example, between not being able to retrieve information and not being able to recognize it from choices.

Language Profile

Progressive impairment in language functioning due to neurodegenerative brain disease, also known as PPA, typically presents with trouble thinking of words in conversation, understanding the meaning of words, problems writing, and mistakes in grammar when speaking and/or writing.[17] The aphasia is caused by dysfunction of the perisylvian region in the language dominant (usually left) hemisphere of the brain. Neuropsychologists and/or speech-language pathologists assess language functioning by having the individual complete tests that assess the ability to name objects, repeat words, point to objects that are named, read, write, execute commands, and quickly list words related to a cue, such as a specific category (eg, animals) or a specific letter (eg, the letter "F"). They also test an individual's ability to understand the meaning of single words and grammatically simple and complex sentences.

Visuospatial Profile

Visuospatial and other types of visual perceptual changes occur when the brain loses its ability to "make sense" of visual information in the environment. These changes are not due to problems with visual acuity, or "eyesight," but, instead, individuals with this disorder have difficulty scanning the environment in an informative manner and paying attention to salient information in the periphery or even in the central field of vision. This syndrome, also referred to as PCA,[13] is associated with degeneration in the occipito-parietal and temporoparietal areas of the brain,[18,19] regions implicated in the interpretation of the nature of visual stimuli and their locations. Neuropsychologists assess visuospatial and perceptual abilities by asking an individual to search for shapes or letters on a page containing many target and nontarget stimuli, draw and copy geometric designs, complete visual puzzles, or estimate angles.

Behavior/Comportment Profile

Changes in behavior and personality are noticeable when an individual acts or behaves uncharacteristically. For example, the once kind and polite individual becomes rude and makes inappropriate comments, violating social norms. Conversely, someone who was always outgoing and gregarious becomes placid and lacks initiative. Sometimes abnormal behaviors are an exaggeration of preexisting personality traits. Research diagnostic criteria have been proposed and validated for this syndrome, which is referred to as bvFTD.[12,20] Abnormal behaviors and personality changes arise from frontal network dysfunction. This network regulates emotional reactivity, judgment, and social conduct. Early symptoms in daily life include impaired judgment, perseverating on certain topics, apathy, social disinhibition, impulsivity, and changes in usual emotional reactions (eg, loss of empathy and sympathy). The key to making a diagnosis is not only whether or not a symptom is present but also if it represents a change from a prior customary state.

Additional Psychiatric and Neurologic Symptoms Considered for the Care Pathway Model for Dementia

Dementia can be accompanied by motor symptoms in several types of disease, including motor neuron disease (amyotrophic lateral sclerosis), corticobasal syndrome, progressive supranuclear palsy, and cortical Lewy body disease (LBD). Vascular cognitive impairment caused by cerebrovascular disease can also be associated with motor symptoms. These symptoms reflect that the disease is affecting systems involved with motor coordination, speed, and planning of movement and complex sequences of actions. If motor symptoms exist, care recommendations can include physical and occupational therapy.

Depression and other affective symptoms are known to be present in individuals diagnosed with DAT, PPA,[21] and other dementia syndromes[22] and can have a negative impact on activities of daily living, progression of disease, and quality of life.[23] Affective symptoms can have a significant impact on the implementation of strategies and interventions and need to be considered when making recommendations to patients and caregivers. Mood and other psychiatric symptoms can be assessed by interviewing patients or their caregivers and having them respond to self-report questionnaires, such as the Geriatric Depression Scale[24] or the brief questionnaire form of the Neuropsychiatric Inventory[25]

Some patients may also have disorders of sleep, particularly if the underlying cause is LBD.[26] Sleep disorders can often lead to worsening of symptoms during waking hours and are also disruptive to caregivers who may be awakened during the night or, conversely, may have difficulty if a patient falls asleep often during the day. Sleep disorders should be evaluated because treatment may improve quality of life.

THE PSYCHOSOCIAL ASSESSMENT

After a neurocognitive assessment, patients are referred to social workers for a psychosocial assessment, which is an evaluation of a patient and family's mental, physical, and emotional health. Usually, a psychosocial assessment is obtained in a conversational interview with the patient and family to assess how individuals and their families are coping with the illness; their familial and other historical relationships; their emotional, social, and financial resources; and overall strengths and challenges. The psychosocial assessment allows for a holistic understanding of how patients and families are living with dementia symptoms, what resources are needed, and their capacity to reorganize themselves around the changes that the illness brings (and will continue to bring) to their lives.

The psychosocial assessment engages the family in a trusting working relationship to learn how a patient and family view the "problem" in their words. How well do the individual and family understand the symptoms and the connection between symptoms and the diagnosis? How are the cognitive symptoms specifically affecting the person's life and what effects do these changes have on the family? How do memory loss, aphasia, visuospatial deficits, or behavioral changes affect social relationships, safety, personal interests, and ability to participate in meaningful activities? How do the predominant symptoms specifically interfere with the ability to perform routine daily activities and carry out normal day-to-day responsibilities? How do the symptoms affect their mood? What symptoms are identified by the person with dementia and their family as most concerning?

Personal, familial, socioeconomic, community, and cultural influences on the patient and family are also addressed. For example, how is the family as a whole managing and coping? What is most challenging and what financial, emotional, and social resources do they have available over the course of the illness? An understanding of the family's past relational functioning influences how they experience current changes.

The psychological, social, family, and financial issues that affect individuals with young-onset dementia are very different from those that affect individuals with late-onset dementia. Not only are the patients younger but also their families are younger. Job-related tasks cannot be performed when patients find it difficult to carry on conversations or control inconsiderate behaviors or when they are increasingly forgetful. Employers and coworkers do not understand why an individual is having difficulty. Individuals are at risk of receiving poor performance evaluations, bringing a loss of self-esteem and a feeling of diminished productivity, and may be terminated from their positions before the illness is understood or diagnosed. Therefore, persons with young-onset dementia who are often still working have to stop working in the prime of their careers when they are saving for retirement and supporting a young family. Because of the loss of employment, a spouse or partner may need to seek additional work to meet the family's financial needs, or other family members, such as siblings and sometimes even parents, step in to offer financial support. The loss of income also has an impact on the affordability of future long-term care. Many have not saved enough yet and may also have young children they are supporting. Living with young-onset dementia is a defining experience for the entire family. It can have negative and positive ramifications and care must be taken to both understand how everyone is coping and recognize that each person in the family is experiencing the illness in his or her own way.

INTERVENTION STRATEGIES

Outcomes from the neurocognitive and psychosocial assessments are used to identify the most appropriate care pathway for a patient's specific symptoms. Interventions in CARE-D take a holistic approach to address functional impairments that focus on increasing an individual's participation in meaningful, productive activities throughout the course of the disease while maintaining dignity at all times. Cognitive retraining and introduction to compensatory strategies are targeted in the early stages; environmental modifications and compensatory strategies are emphasized in the later stages. Ongoing family/caregiver education and training to promote generalization and implementation of strategies is essential throughout all stages. Home safety and driving evaluations are necessary components of each care pathway. For each care pathway, it is also important to assess an individual's hobbies and interests, motivation, and awareness of deficits as well as the level of caregiver involvement and support.

Memory Care Pathway

The goal of the memory care pathway is to compensate for the inability to retain information and enable an individual to maintain independence through use of external memory aids, memory devices, and environmental modifications. Strategies also aim to reduce frustration and stress using techniques that not only maximize maintaining a routine, structure, and consistency but also provide safety in areas where forgetfulness could result in financial or personal jeopardy. If spontaneous retrieval is impaired but recognition memory is relatively preserved, strategies could use cues/triggers to aid recall. Specific interventions are provided in **Table 1**. Speech-language pathologists and occupational therapists are best suited to identify appropriate practical strategies for each family.

Language Care Pathway

Strategies for the language care pathway aim to support communication with the affected individual by offering education and communication tips for family members and augmentative communication methods so that a person with dementia can maintain independence in daily activities. A combination of impairment-directed interventions that are focused on enhancing a particular area of deficiency (eg, improving motor sequencing for patients with apraxia of speech) and activity/participation-based interventions that are focused on the patient participating in a particular action or activity in daily life (eg, training a patient to use an augmentative and alternate communication device to help participate in a conversation)[27] are often appropriate, with frequent adjustments to the recommended strategies to meet an individual's changing communication needs as the disease progresses. Interventions should focus on personally relevant stimuli to generalize to functional contexts as much as possible (see **Table 1** for example strategies).[28–30] A speech-language pathologist is the most relevant referral for this pathway.

Visuospatial Care Pathway

For those individuals experiencing perceptual or visuospatial deficits, the goal of the visuospatial care pathway is to modify the home environment to accommodate these changes and incorporate the use of technology to improve safety and independence. **Table 1** provides examples of environmental and technological modifications that are often used by occupational therapists. In addition to referrals to an occupational therapist, specialized services for individuals with low vision may be useful, even though the main obstacle is not visual acuity.

Behavior Care Pathway

The goal of the behavior care pathway is to maximize safety for a person with dementia who lacks judgment and decision-making ability and to minimize the stress of family members involved in the care by replacing confrontation with alternative responses to behavior changes (see **Table 1** for example strategies).[30] Many of the strategies for this pathway require implementation by family members rather than the affected individual who often lacks the initiative to follow instructions. Psychiatrists and social workers are most commonly consulted but speech-language pathologists and occupational therapists may contribute by providing recommendations for home safety and assessing the amount of supervision needed at home and in the community.

PROCEDURES OF THE CARE PATHWAY PROGRAM

The CARE-D program grew out of a seed grant obtained in 2010 to pilot test the role of a Care Pathway Resource Coordinator to connect individual clinic patients and families with services and maintain communication among all involved. The experience

Table 1
Four care pathways for dementia: common neuropsychological profiles, deficits in daily living activities, and strategies and interventions

Common Neurocognitive Findings	Common Symptoms in Daily Living Reflecting Primary Deficit	Common Strategies/Interventions
Memory Dementia Care Pathway		
Poor orientation to time and place	Mixes up appointments; takes medications at the wrong times or completely forgets them; does not know the day, date, and, when more advanced, time of day	Spaced retrieval training (ie, gradually increasing recall intervals to promote learning)[37,38]
Acquisition deficits: scores are low on tests of learning words, stories, and designs, and, despite repeated trials, cannot increase the amount of information recalled	Despite repeated information/instructions, cannot retain information; may ask the same question over and over again within a short interval of time	Errorless learning: learning that occurs in a facilitated environment that eliminates errors[39]
Retention and retrieval deficits: after a delay even as brief as 3 min, cannot recall the information initially learned	Information evaporates and patients may argue that they were never told the information	Vanishing cues hierarchy: the systematic reduction of cue information across learning trials[40]
Performance does not improve with multiple-choice recognition and the patient may also "recognize" information that was not previously presented (ie, make false-positive identifications)	Cannot use cues to remember; seeing a familiar landmark does not remind the patient of location or direction to move in	Use of memory wallets/books to promote recall of orientation facts, important names, past and recent events, and other functional facts, such as safety precautions[41]
		External or electronic memory aids, such as schedule boards[42,43]
		Environmental modifications to improve participation in activities of daily living and safety (eg, lighting, flooring, color schemes, wall hangings, furniture, and noise/sound)
		Ongoing training of caregivers/family members on the use of positive communication strategies and the importance of avoiding questions that rely on short-term memory also contributes to a reduction in difficult behaviors[44]
		Safety devices, such as GPS personal locator devices, home monitor device, adaptive telephones, identification bracelets

Language Dementia Care Pathway

Low scores on tests of object naming; makes errors (may say "microscope" instead of "stethoscope") May not understand single words even when they are common (eg, asking "What is salt?") or sentences that are grammatically complex (eg, "Who is the boy that John kicked?") Low scores on tests of reading comprehension and writing	Gropes for words so that speech is interrupted by long pauses for word-finding Cannot carry out instructions; may misunderstand what is being said, despite normal hearing, and misinterpret messages, which can lead to anger and even paranoia Cannot understand written communications (newspapers, books); cannot write normally; makes errors in spelling and/or grammar	Self-cueing strategies (eg, semantic circumlocution) Home exercise program targeting the rehearsal of personally relevant words Oral reading tasks, including strategies to increase motor sequencing for multisyllabic words (eg, syllabic segmentation, Melodic Intonation Therapy)[45] Personal picture description tasks Script rehearsal for telephone conversations and in social contexts Communication tools to supplement spoken language as the disease progresses include use of a communication wallet, communication boards/book, and possibly an augmentative and alternate communication device[29,46] Strategies to help an individual compensate for dyslexia and dysgraphia, including technology that provides auditory and visual cues to promote reading comprehension; for dysgraphia, speech recognition apps and word prediction features can help facilitate functional writing tasks

(*continued on next page*)

Table 1
(continued)

Common Neurocognitive Findings	Common Symptoms in Daily Living Reflecting Primary Deficit	Common Strategies/Interventions
Visuospatial Dementia Care Pathway		
Low scores on tests requiring spatial perception, such as deciding if 2 lines are at the same angle as a model	Misjudging distance and relationship of body to external space, which can result in car accidents or scrapes when trying to park or pass between fences	Environmental modifications: increasing organization around the home, decreasing clutter, using proper lighting, controlling glare, and increasing contrast
Difficulty finding specific targets on a sheet containing many different types of letters or shapes; search strategy is unsystematic and patient may miss many targets despite normal visual acuity	Difficulty searching for household items; items may be in plain view and, especially if surrounded by other items (as an item in a drawer or in a refrigerator), are "invisible" to the patient	Use of technology for compensation: talking watches/alarm clocks, a large numbered phone, a reading machine, a magnifier with a light feature, and a variety of voice-activated enabled smartphones
Difficulty drawing a clock or copying a simple geometric figure; difficulty putting blocks together to make a visual pattern	Inability to place objects on a table surface; difficulty assembling kitchen utensils; difficulty orienting clothing to one's body or working knobs and accessories in the car	Reduce the size of print for individuals with simultanagnosia
Facial discrimination problems and inability to decide if 2 faces seen from different perspectives are the same person or not	Misrecognizing people; not able to easily recognize facial differences	
	Larger letters can be more difficult to recognize due to "simultanagnosia"	
Behavior Dementia Care Pathway		
Has difficulty reasoning and performing cognitive shifting tasks	Makes poor decisions, which may jeopardize financial or personal safety or the safety of others; thinking is rigid; cannot come up with or understand alternative solutions to problems	Communication tips or visual cue strategies to best respond to behavioral changes, such as agitation disinhibition, poor judgment, etc.[47]
Loses knowledge about what is socially acceptable in different settings	Engages in embarrassing behaviors (eg, talking loud or laughing during a funeral service); makes insulting remarks; sloppy eating habits	Emotional support and respite care for the primary caregiver
Cannot inhibit automatic responses	May unintentionally engage in criminal behavior (eg, "shoplifting"); touches objects; may dial the phone just because it is there	Safety devices, such as GPS personal locator devices, home monitor device, adaptive telephones, identification bracelets
May incorporate stimuli irrelevant to the task at hand because they are accessible, known as stimulus-bound behavior		

Memory dementia care pathway

Betty (age 62) was given a clinical diagnosis of DAT 2 years earlier. Bill, to whom Betty had been married 35 years, continued to work full time in the family business. Their 3 daughters lived nearby and tried to spend a lot of time with her but had a difficult time knowing what might be most helpful for their mother and were torn between helping their mother and caring for their own school-age children. Betty worked as a grade school teacher until it became too difficult to manage her lesson plans. She enjoyed learning new skills through adult learning classes in her community. She attended Catholic Mass every Sunday. Neuropsychological examination was completed and episodic memory was the primary problem, with other domains either normal or less impaired than memory. For example, on the Repeatable Battery for the Assessment of Neuropsychological Status Update,[31] she was able to learn 8 of 10 words on the list learning subtest but after a brief delay could recall only 2 and could not recognize all the words on multiple choice. In contrast, she had no difficulty copying a complex figure, her digit span was 8 forward and 6 backward, and she was able to achieve a normal number of categories on the Wisconsin Card Sorting Test (WCST).[32] Practical interventions were aimed at providing supports for impaired short-term memory.

Psychosocial assessment established that Betty was frustrated with being forced to give up driving. Her increased dependency on her family was straining her relationships with her husband and her daughters as she attempted to hold on to as much independence as possible. Reciprocally, her daughters did not know how much to assist their mother and what they could allow her to do safely. Helping Betty maintain her independence by focusing on her remaining strengths and identifying helpful strategies to compensate for changes helped reduce her frustration and stress. Psychosocial interventions of counseling and education helped the family know when to step in to help, when to step back and support Betty's autonomy, and how to balance their mother's needs with those of their children and identify and address their own emotional needs for self-care. **Table 2** *delineates the symptoms, strengths, and recommendations for this pathway.*

Language dementia care pathway

Margaret (age 52) was diagnosed with PPA 3 years earlier. She obtained a PhD in education and, after a career of teaching at the university level, she became dean at a local college. Margaret was forced to stop working when communication problems began to interfere with her ability to deliver her classroom lectures and interact with her colleagues. She also had difficulty finishing a book that she started writing a few years earlier. Margaret, with her partner of 23 years, had 2 sons, ages 10 and 12. Her interests included reading biographies and traveling. Margaret's partner worked full time.

Neuropsychological testing found language the primary problem. Although Margaret could understand single words, she had difficulty when presented with complex grammatical constructions and multistep commands. She also had significant difficulty naming objects. On the Boston Naming Test,[33] she scored 35 of a possible 60. Her errors indicated that she recognized the objects but had difficulty retrieving the words without a phonemic cue. Finally, word-finding difficulty was also evident in spontaneous speech. When trying to tell the "Picnic" story from the Western Aphasia Battery-Revised,[34] she had frequent hesitations before nouns and often provided circumlocution for words she could not retrieve.

The psychosocial assessment brought to light a close supportive relationship between Margaret and her partner who adjusted his work life as a journalist to accommodate her increasing needs and to focus on the care of their 2 children. Finances were a major concern. An application was submitted for Social Security Disability Insurance and they consulted with an elder law attorney for estate planning. Margaret's awareness of her declining abilities contributed to her depressed mood, and her partner, although supportive, expressed much grief at the losses they were enduring as a family. Disclosing the diagnosis to their young sons was aided by consulting the Association for Frontotemporal Degeneration's specialized resources (www. aftdkidsandteens.org). The goal of CARE-D intervention was to support Margaret's communication and enhance mood by offering education and communication strategies for her family. The program also provided methods for Margaret to maintain independence in daily activities and engage in meaningful activities. *Table 3* identifies symptoms, strengths, and CARE-D recommendations for Margaret.

Visuospatial dementia care pathway

Steve (age 57) was diagnosed 2 months earlier with visuospatial dysfunction (PCA). Steve lived with his spouse of 25 years in their home. His spouse worked a demanding full-time job at the peak of her career. They had 1 adopted daughter, who was married with a newborn child. Neuropsychological testing found visual perception as the primary problem. Visual target search was erratic and he missed many items on both sides of the page. Constructions were severely impaired and he was unable to complete the Trail Making Tests due to difficulty visually locating the appropriate next item, even though he had not lost his sequencing ability. In contrast, despite difficulty initially acquiring a list of words, he was able to retain the amount he initially learned after a delay. In daily life, the words seemed to "jump off the page" while reading, he had difficulty accurately reaching for objects, and driving became harrowing due to his problems with depth perception and getting lost. Steve also began having difficulty navigating his home as the illness began to eventually affect gait and balance.

An in-depth psychosocial evaluation revealed that Steve and his wife had experienced a troubled relationship on and off throughout their marriage. Steve's wife resented his increasing dependence on her, because this interfered with her demanding workload. Steve called his wife several times during the day because he had more trouble navigating his world independently. Steve's wife admitted that she feared that her goals of achieving a higher-level position, in the work that she loved, would be compromised by the illness because Steve required so much of her attention. Fortunately, Steve and his wife had a long-term care insurance policy that allowed her to hire care at home while she worked. This helped relieve some of the stress she experienced, and she sought counseling and participated in a support group to help manage her feelings of anger and grief. Occupational therapy recommendations for changes in Steve's home environment helped accommodate visuospatial deficits and improve his safety and independence. *Table 4* identifies Steve's symptoms, strengths, and CARE-D recommendations.

Behavior dementia care pathway

Sam (age 61) was diagnosed with bvFTD 4 years earlier. Ruth, who is Sam's wife of 23 years, worked full time as a journalist. Her daughter from her previous marriage lived nearby. Sam had 2 adult children from a previous marriage; however, they were estranged. Sam was a law professor for 30 years, until he was forced to retire due to his symptoms. Sam used to be active in his community through a civic club and politics but had not been involved in these activities for the past 10 years. Neuropsychological testing identified that reasoning and comportment were Sam's primary areas of difficulty. Although Sam's scores on tests of episodic memory and even on the executive attention test, Trail Making Test, Part B, were normal, on the WCST he had difficulty with mental flexibility and switching from one category to another. Ruth identified significant changes on the Frontal Systems Behavioral Scale,[35] including disinhibition, which was not part of his personality in the past. In addition, he also had signs of increasing executive dysfunction and apathy in daily life. Practical interventions were based on addressing obstreperous behaviors and maintaining a regular schedule.

Psychosocial assessment revealed that Sam's increased apathy over several years and misdiagnosis of his illness had led his wife to consider divorce. She expressed being overwhelmed and confused regarding how to respond to her husband's lack of emotion for her, in addition to the grief over the loss of their close relationship and dreams for the future. Interventions focused on maximizing Sam's safety and helping Ruth learn communication strategies while minimizing the daily stress she experienced. *Table 5* delineates the symptoms, strengths, and recommendations.

Table 2
Memory dementia care pathway vignette

How Memory Loss is Affecting Betty's Daily Life	Betty's Identified Strengths	Corresponding Recommendations for Betty
Misplacing items	Visuospatial function intact	Implemented a system at home where the most important items (cell phone, purse, keys, etc.) are left in one well-marked spot in the house. A home occupational therapy consultation was ordered to focus on memory and organizational strategies to reduce clutter and to create systems for better organization of personal belongings, paperwork, and bathroom and kitchen items for improved activities of daily living performance.
Forgetting/missing appointments	Able to read	Advised Betty to use a large calendar on which she could write many details about her appointments including time, location, topic, and phone number. Set up a reminder system for her family to check her calendar on a daily basis. Implemented use of a dry-erase board next to the calendar to list times of daily activities and other important reminders. Betty crossed off each day of the calendar as it passed, using a clock next to the calendar that displayed the time and date.
Withdrawing from activities, including reading and socializing with friends	Only minor problems with language functioning	Modified activities, which do not rely on memory but fit Betty's interests, including water aerobics and using a computer with a visual memory aid displaying a picture and short description for each step for checking and sending e-mails. Referral made to speech-language therapy at home to help formulate visual memory aids. Family trained to assist Betty with writing down 2 stimulating activities per day on her dry-erase board. Audio and visual reminders set up by family on her phone to increase initiation of the selected activities.

Table 3
Language dementia care pathway vignette

How the Aphasia is Affecting Margaret's Daily Life	Margaret's Identified Strengths	Corresponding Recommendations for Margaret
Margaret is less active socially and finds it hard to stay busy when her partner is at work. She often watches TV and wishes she had more to do.	She is independent in most of her personal activities of daily living.	New modified community activities were suggested, including volunteer work that does not rely heavily on communication with others, such as walking dogs for a local shelter.
Margaret has word finding pauses and hesitations and increased difficulty with auditory comprehension at the conversation level. Spontaneous speech is especially difficult when speaking over the telephone.	Margaret has preserved memory for recent events; no behavioral changes have been reported.	Create a communication friendly environment by reducing distractions, using one-on-one conversations and speaking in simple sentences to facilitate auditory comprehension. Communication enhancement strategies (eg, family asking more "yes-no" questions and Margaret using gestures to help explain what she is trying to say). Speech therapy focused on creating home program targeting the rehearsal of personally relevant words, including names, important locations, and other important words she uses during daily conversations. Telephone scripts were designed and rehearsed to promote word retrieval and fluency during telephone conversations.
Her partner and children are less likely to converse with her for fear of creating frustrating situations when she cannot find a word.	She has preserved insight into her condition and resulting changes.	Speech-language pathologist trained Margaret and her family to create a system for when to help fill in the words for her during conversation. Also trained family on appropriate verbal cues to increase Margaret's use of semantic circumlocution, so she can self-cue or communicate her message more easily to others. A communication wallet was also created, which contains lists of words by category that Margaret frequently uses during conversations with family and friends. Margaret was trained to use the wallet when unable to retrieve the word. Education on the disease and support was provided for her young sons and her partner. Directed family to the Association for Frontotemporal Dementia Web site for kids and teens http://www.aftdkidsandteens.org.
Errors with spelling	She is interested in writing e-mails to friends and family.	Used augmentative technology, such as the Google application or Dragon software on Margaret's smartphone to assist her with spelling. With this application, she could speak the word and the device used speech recognition software to spell out the word for her.

Table 4
Visuospatial dementia care pathway vignette

How the Visuospatial Perceptual Deficits are Affecting Steve's Daily Life	Steve's Identified Strengths	Corresponding Recommendations for Steve
Steve enjoyed an active social life but lately has withdrawn from socializing with others due to impaired driving ability.	He maintains an interest in socializing with friends and he has no problems with verbal communication.	New modified community activities that do not rely on Steve's visual perception, such as attending art- and music-based activities and programs in the community accompanied by a companion so he does not need to drive.
Steve is having difficulty writing and using a calendar.	He has only minor problems with short-term memory and no other cognitive impairments at this time.	Referral to an occupational therapist to increase use of compensatory strategies for schedule management, including selection of visually simple calendar, use of highlighting and color coding, and use of block lettering with space in between each letter. A large display clock with the time and date was recommended.
Due to his visual changes, there are safety risks for activities within his home including cooking, ironing, and driving.	Steve is independent in all his personal activities of daily living.	Introduced environmental changes, including the use of bright lights, decluttering, and removing throw rugs to decrease falls. In the kitchen Steve was encouraged to use labels to help him find objects and organize the refrigerator so that he could find objects based on location (eg, "second shelf") if he could not "see" them. The occupational therapist also reviewed safety issues at home with Steve's wife.
He walks more slowly and hesitates when on sidewalks with curbs and while using stairs.	Steve is physically strong and has good balance.	Referral to a local low vision support program for additional services to accommodate visual changes.

from this initial trial resulted in reconfiguring the model not to create a bottleneck for services but to implement a clinic procedure in which all clinicians participate. After the clinical evaluation, typically neurologic and neuropsychological examinations, a patient is discussed at weekly clinic management rounds attended by speech and occupational therapists and social workers. A list of needed professionals is

Table 5
Behavior dementia care pathway vignette

How the Behavioral Deficits are Affecting Sam's Daily Life	Sam's Identified Strengths	Corresponding Recommendations for Sam
Fixating on topics for long periods of time	Enjoys wood working	Communication strategies were provided for Sam's wife; for example, using distraction when Sam fixates on topics. During the appointment, Sam's wife and a therapist role-played this strategy using the example of refocusing Sam's attention to an enjoyable activity, such as woodworking. Written cues in a memory wallet were also introduced to decrease perseveration on topics and to increase initiation of meaningful questions during conversations with family members.
Taking an extended time dressing and getting ready in the morning due to changes in initiation	Can follow simple written instructions	Step-by-step instructions with images to help Sam get ready in the morning were designed to assist Sam with brushing his teeth and hair. A referral was made to speech-language therapy in the home to help formulate these visual memory aids.
Problems with motivation and making decisions	Performs well with structured routine and participates in some household work	A daily schedule of activities was created so that Sam was not faced with decisions and was offered structure. Activities were written on a dry-erase schedule board to increase recall of past/upcoming activities. Activities focused on his interests in a modified and simplified way. For example, instead of using the woodworking equipment, Sam spent time sanding various pieces of wood for a project that his friend later helped him put together.
Makes inappropriate comments to strangers that are embarrassing to his wife		Sam's wife was counseled on strategies to help her cope with Sam's disinhibition. These included disclosing the diagnosis to close friends and family to increase their awareness and, as much as possible, avoiding public situations where Sam's behavior could be particularly troubling to her. Sam's wife was also given a card that she could show to strangers briefly explaining Sam's diagnosis and asking for their patience and understanding. Sam was referred to a behavioral home health program and a psychiatrist to assist with managing behavior changes. Sam's wife was referred to a frontotemporal dementia caregiver support group to help her cope with Sam's changes as well as help guide her with long-term planning.
Frequent irritability		The social worker explored and identified triggers for Sam's irritability and counseled family on interventions that may help to avoid these symptoms, such as playing calming music and remaining nonconfrontational.

generated and the patient is referred directly to the one(s) identified as most central in the care pathway. All patients and families are also referred to social work. Continuity of care is maintained through medical record communication and feedback at the weekly meetings about how the care plan is proceeding and if any changes are needed. The ability for the clinicians and care providers to communicate efficiently with one another is a sine qua non of this program.

Costs are reimbursable by Medicare Part B and other insurance providers as part of a person's care plan. Speech and occupational therapies are provided both at home and in the outpatient clinical setting based on the specific needs of the individual and family.

The interdisciplinary nature of the CARE-D model, what is believed to be its success, requires increased attention be paid to the clinical training and education received in dementia not only within schools of medicine but also within schools of speech, occupational therapies, social work, and other allied health professions who come into contact with persons with dementia and have the opportunity to contribute to their optimal level of functioning throughout the course of the illness. Recognizing the need of these professions for specialized dementia education, the Northwestern clinical team is committed to continuing education and training of those with whom we work to provide optimal care and treatment. For example, in collaboration with the Association for Frontotemporal Degeneration and the National Aphasia Association, a 3-part webinar series on PPA and other clinical dementia syndromes for speech-language pathologists was designed and implemented[36] and is accessible free of charge (http://www.brain.northwestern.edu/about/events/webinar.html). Another helpful source is the International PPA Connection Web site (http://www.ppaconnection.org), which provides resources and support for clinicians, researchers, patients, and family members.

DISCUSSION

CARE-D builds a tailored care plan based on data from an individual's psychosocial and neuropsychological assessments. The psychosocial context is an essential component and consideration is given to patients' and families' living situations, social support systems, life stages, financial resources, and understanding of their preexisting coping strategies and historical relationships. This ensures that the recommendations are realistic for families, from both psychological and practical perspectives. For an individual who has dementia, the interventions focus on the person's abilities and strengths. The introduction of tailored interventions and activities may allow family and friends to focus more on their relationship with the person as a spouse/partner, adult child, sibling, or friend rather than their role as a caregiver. The ultimate goal is to enhance quality of life for all as they significantly restructure their lives to cope with an individual's progressive disability.

The CARE-D model relies on a skilled interdisciplinary team to be successful. The evaluation by a neuropsychologist to establish the neurocognitive profile and symptoms as well as remaining strengths is vital to establishing the interventions. The CARE-D model has been developed in close collaboration with speech and occupational therapists knowledgeable about dementia and the neurodegenerative nature of the illness, who focus on compensatory strategies and remaining abilities. Thus, persons with dementia and their families are provided with helpful methods to manage the changes and contribute to a better quality of life. Understanding the strengths of the family, their relationships, and the context in which they are able to cope with and implement the proposed recommendations informs the team of what challenges the family is facing and what psychosocial support is needed to help sustain the family over time.

Finally, for this model to have wider replication in other clinic and primary care settings, research is needed to quantify and identify measureable outcomes. There is the potential for this model to have an impact on the larger health care system. By making recommendations that target symptom-specific profiles, disease stage, and life stage and focus on remaining strengths, this approach to care may help reduce unnecessary health care costs associated with improper/inadequate care, reduce hospitalizations, and delay long-term care placement. The model recognizes the complexity of dementia syndromes and the unique needs of each person with dementia and the families. This is particularly important because dementia is being diagnosed at earlier stages than in the past, at a time when cognitive impairments may be isolated to 1 or 2 cognitive and/or behavioral domains and may remain that way for several years prior to more generalized impairment.

REFERENCES

1. Alzheimer's Association. Early-onset dementia: a national challenge, a future crisis. Washington, DC: Alzheimer's Association; 2006.
2. McKhann GM, Albert MS, Grossman M, et al. Clinical and pathological diagnosis of frontotemporal dementia. Arch Neurol 2001;58:1803–9.
3. Weintraub S, Mesulam MM. Four neuropsychological profiles in dementia. In: Boller F, Grafman J, editors. Handbook of neuropsychology. Amsterdam: Elsevier; 1993. p. 253–81.
4. Price BH, Gurvit H, Weintraub S, et al. Neuropsychological patterns and language deficits in 20 consecutive cases of autopsy-confirmed Alzheimer's disease. Arch Neurol 1993;50:931–7.
5. Freyne A, Kidd N, Coen R, et al. Burden in carers of dementia patients: higher levels in carers of younger sufferers. Int J Geriatr Psychiatry 1999;14:784–8.
6. Gitlin LN, Winter L, Vause Earland T, et al. The Tailored Activity Program to reduce behavioral symptoms in individuals with dementia: feasibility, acceptability, and replication potential. Gerontologist 2009;49:428–39.
7. Weintraub S, Morhardt D. Treatment, education, and resources for non-alzheimer dementia: one size does not fit all. Alzheimer's Care Today 2005;6:201–14.
8. Weintraub S. Neuropsychological assessment of dementia: a large-scale neuroanatomical network approach. In: Dickerson BC, Atri A, editors. Dementia: comprehensive principles and practice. New York: Oxford University Press; 2014. p. 487–507.
9. Weintraub S, Mesulam MM. From neuronal networks to dementia: four clinical profiles. In: Foret F, Christen Y, Boller F, editors. La Demence: Pourquoi? Paris: Foundation Nationale de Gerontologie; 1996. p. 75–97.
10. Weintraub S, Rubin NP, Mesulam MM. Primary progressive aphasia. Longitudinal course, neuropsychological profile, and language features. Arch Neurol 1990;47: 1329–35.
11. McKhann GM, Knopman DS, Chertkow H, et al. The diagnosis of dementia due to Alzheimer's disease: recommendations from the National Institute on Aging-Alzheimer's Association workgroups on diagnostic guidelines for Alzheimer's disease. Alzheimers Dement 2011;7:263–9.
12. Rascovsky K, Hodges JR, Kipps CM, et al. Diagnostic criteria for the behavioral variant of frontotemporal dementia (bvFTD): current limitations and future directions. Alzheimer Dis Assoc Disord 2007;21:S14–8.

13. Benson DF, Davis RJ, Snyder BD. Posterior cortical atrophy. Arch Neurol 1988;45: 789–93.
14. Gorno-Tempini ML, Hillis AE, Weintraub S, et al. Classification of primary progressive aphasia and its variants. Neurology 2011;76:1006–14.
15. Squire LR. Memory systems of the brain: a brief history and current perspective. Neurobiol Learn Mem 2004;82:171–7.
16. Mesulam MM. Neuroplasticity failure in Alzheimer's disease: bridging the gap between plaques and tangles. Neuron 1999;24:521–9.
17. Mesulam MM. Primary progressive aphasia. Ann Neurol 2001;49:425–32.
18. Mendez MF, Perryman KM. Neuropsychiatric features of frontotemporal dementia: evaluation of consensus criteria and review. J Neuropsychiatry Clin Neurosci 2002;14:424–9.
19. Renner JA, Burns JM, Hou CE, et al. Progressive posterior cortical dysfunction: a clinicopathologic series. Neurology 2004;63:1175–80.
20. Rascovsky K, Hodges JR, Knopman D, et al. Sensitivity of revised diagnostic criteria for the behavioural variant of frontotemporal dementia. Brain 2011;134: 2456–77.
21. Medina J, Weintraub S. Depression in primary progressive aphasia. J Geriatr Psychiatry Neurol 2007;20:153–60.
22. Ballard C, Patel A, Oyebode F, et al. Cognitive decline in patients with Alzheimer's disease, vascular dementia and senile dementia of Lewy body type. Age Ageing 1996;25:209–13.
23. Lyketsos CG, Steele C, Baker L, et al. Major and minor depression in Alzheimer's disease: prevalence and impact. J Neuropsychiatry Clin Neurosci 1997;9: 556–61.
24. Yesavage JA, Brink TL, Rose TL, et al. Development and validation of a geriatric depression screening scale: a preliminary report. J Psychiatr Res 1982;17: 37–49.
25. Kaufer DI, Cummings JL, Ketchel P, et al. Validation of the NPI-Q, a brief clinical form of the Neuropsychiatric Inventory. J Neuropsychiatry Clin Neurosci 2000;12: 233–9.
26. Ferman TJ, Boeve BF, Smith GE, et al. REM sleep behavior disorder and dementia: cognitive differences when compared with AD. Neurology 1999;52:951–7.
27. Croot K, Nickels L, Laurence F, et al. Impairment- and activity/participation-directed interventions in progressive language impairment: clinical and theoretical issues. Aphasiology 2009;23:125–60.
28. Khayum B, Wieneke C, Rogalski E, et al. Thinking outside the stroke: treating Primary Progressive Aphasia (PPA). Perspect Gerontol 2012;17(2):37–49.
29. Taylor C, Kingma RM, Croot K, et al. Speech pathology services for primary progressive aphasia: exploring an emerging area of practice. Aphasiology 2009;23: 161–74.
30. Kortte KB, Rogalski EJ. Behavioural interventions for enhancing life participation in behavioural variant frontotemporal dementia and primary progressive aphasia. Int Rev Psychiatry 2013;25:237–45.
31. Randolph C. Repeatable battery for the assessment of neuropsychological status update. San Antonio (TX): Pearson; 2012.
32. Heaton RK. Wisconsin card sorting test (WCST) manual revised and expanded. Odessa (FL): Psychological Assessment Resources; 1993.
33. Goodglass H, Kaplan E, Weintraub S. Boston naming test. Philadelphia: Lea & Febiger; 1983.
34. Kertesz A. Western aphasia battery - revised (WAB-R). Austin (TX): Pro-Ed; 2006.

35. Grace J, Mallory PF. Frontal systems behavioral scale professional manual. Lutz, FL: Psychological Assessment Resources Inc; 2001.
36. Ganzfried E, Morhardt D, Denny S. The SLP & Primary Progressive Aphasia (PPA): developing an education coalition. Chicago: American Speech and Hearing Association Annual Convention; 2013.
37. Camp CJ. Spaced retrieval: a model for dissemination of a cognitive intervention for persons with dementia. In: Attix DK, Welsh-Bohmer KA, editors. Geriatric neuropsychology: assessment and intervention. New York: The Guilford Press; 2006. p. 275–92.
38. Hopper T, Bourgeois M, Pimentel J, et al. An evidence-based systematic review on cognitive interventions for individuals with dementia. Am J Speech Lang Pathol 2013;22:126–45.
39. Clare L, Jones RS. Errorless learning in the rehabilitation of memory impairment: a critical review. Neuropsychol Rev 2008;18:1–23.
40. Glisky EL, Schacter DL, Tulving E. Learning and retention of computer-related vocabulary in memory-impaired patients: method of vanishing cues. J Clin Exp Neuropsychol 1986;8:292–312.
41. Bourgeois MS, Camp C, Rose M, et al. A comparison of training strategies to enhance use of external aids by persons with dementia. J Commun Disord 2003;36:361–78.
42. Oriani M, Moniz-Cook E, Binetti G, et al. An electronic memory aid to support prospective memory in patients in the early stages of Alzheimer's disease: a pilot study. Aging Ment Health 2003;7:22–7.
43. Lancioni GE, Singh NN, O'Reilly MF, et al. Technology-aided verbal instructions to help persons with mild or moderate Alzheimer's disease perform daily activities. Res Dev Disabil 2010;31:1240–50.
44. Egan M, Berube D, Racine G, et al. Methods to enhance verbal communication between individuals with Alzheimer's disease and their formal and informal caregivers: a systematic review. Int J Alzheimers Dis 2010;2010. http://dx.doi.org/10.4061/2010/906818.
45. Norton A, Zipse L, Marchina S, et al. Melodic Intonation Therapy. Annals of the New York Academy of Sciences 2009;1169:431–6.
46. Beukelman DR, Fager S, Ball L, et al. AAC for adults with acquired neurological conditions: a review. Augment Altern Commun 2007;23:230–42.
47. Logsdon RG, McCurry SM, Teri L. Evidence-based psychological treatments for disruptive behaviors in individuals with dementia. Psychol Aging 2007;22:28–36.

Public Advocacy and Community Engagement
Interventions for Individuals with Young-Onset Dementia and Their Families

Adriana Shnall, PhD, MSW, RSW[a,b,*]

KEYWORDS

- Young-onset dementia • Early-onset dementia • Spousal caregiving
- Dementia caregiving • Psychosocial interventions • Public advocacy
- Community engagement • Family caregiving

KEY POINTS

- There is a lack of tailored services and interventions for those affected by young-onset dementia (YOD). Spouses are the main caregivers and they experience caregiver burden, isolation, depression, and financial difficulties. They have a sense that they are constantly being overlooked by every system (eg, government programs, health care, financial, legal).
- Advocacy is needed to address issues related to the provision of (1) age-appropriate services, (2) adequate in-home supports, (3) changes to the health care system to address their unique needs, and (4) creating suitable policies and financial provisions to support families affected by YOD.
- Interventional studies at the clinical/community level include (1) psychoeducational support groups and (2) respite care in combination with caregiver education and support.
- Proposed areas of intervention for spousal caregivers include leisure activity groups, telephone-based support, and capacity building in the areas of (1) enhancing social supports, (2) financial and legal planning, (3) self-care strategies, and (4) meaningful activities with the patient's spouse.

YOUNG-ONSET DEMENTIA AND ITS EFFECTS ON FAMILIES

Despite the growing awareness of young-onset dementias (YODs), there is a lack of understanding about those living with YOD (both individuals and their families).[1–3]

Disclosure: The author has no relevant or material financial interests that relate to the material presented in this article.
[a] Factor-Inwentash Faculty of Social Work, University of Toronto, 246 Bloor Street W, Toronto, ON M5S1A1, Canada; [b] Sam and Ida Ross Memory Clinic, Baycrest Health Sciences, 3560 Bathurst, ON M6A 2E1, Canada
* Sam and Ida Ross Memory Clinic, Baycrest Health Sciences, 3560 Bathurst, ON M6A 2E1, Canada
E-mail address: ashnall@baycrest.org

Psychiatr Clin N Am 38 (2015) 353–362
http://dx.doi.org/10.1016/j.psc.2015.01.006
0193-953X/15/$ – see front matter © 2015 Elsevier Inc. All rights reserved.

Abbreviations	
LOD	Late-onset dementia
YOD	Young-onset dementia

Knowledge about YOD and its effects on families is necessary for the development of appropriate social and health care interventions. Services for this population are currently inadequate in most countries and most of the dementia services are geared to patients more than 65 years of age.[4] This article highlights the effects of YOD on families, and focuses on public advocacy and community engagement as ways to intervene with patients and their caregivers. Although all family members are affected by having a relative with YOD,[5] spouses/partners of people with YOD are the main caregivers for this group of patients.[2,6,7] Therefore, this article focuses on people with YOD and their spousal caregivers.

Spousal caregivers of younger people with dementia have greater perceived difficulties than those with late-onset dementia (LOD)[4,8–10] and they report greater levels of caregiver burden (eg, the overall physical, emotional, social, and financial costs of caregiving).[11–13] Spousal caregivers in the young-onset group have a higher risk for experiencing loneliness compared with other YOD caregivers such as parents or children.[14] There are multiple financial threats in this group of caregivers: patients lose their employment, spouses may have to cut back or quit their jobs to care for their partners, and patients do not qualify for senior citizen financial and health benefits given their young age.[15,16] Depression is one of the hallmarks of being a spouse of someone with YOD.[10,13,16] The delay in diagnosis (on average, 5 years) adds to the stress of living with someone with YOD.[16,17]

It is important to focus on interventions for families of people with YOD because caregivers' well-being is highly correlated with patients' mental and physical health outcomes.[18–20] Providing tailored supports to families affected by YOD, in particular spousal caregivers, can reduce stress and depression, increase positive aspects of care, and reduce or delay nursing home placement.[18,21] However, there is limited research in the area of YOD and its impact on families and there is no clear understanding on how to best provide services for this group of caregivers.[22] This lack of evidence-based knowledge contributes to a lack of services, which becomes evident when families and health care providers seek care and supports. Professionals are quickly confronted with system issues (eg, lack of financial support, few tailored day programs, nonexistent in-home respite programs), and thus find no feasible solutions to present to families in distress. It is difficult for health care practitioners to deal with the problems that families bring, knowing the dearth of suitable resources. For those affected by YOD, the existing interventions are not sufficient to tackle the problem of lack of resources, and there is no policy targeting the rights and needs of a younger dementia population.[23]

INTERVENTIONS FOR THOSE AFFECTED BY YOUNG-ONSET DEMENTIA
Macro Level of Intervention: Public Advocacy

The health and well-being of families is strongly related to the public policies that are implemented within a society; these are known as the social determinants of health.[24] YOD spousal caregivers are overlooked by the social safety net, creating crises that could be preventable had better social, financial, and health supports been in place.[16] Patients with YOD and their relatives need increased care in the home, flexible respite programs, and placement options that are suitable for their needs. In addition, they require a responsive medical health system and governmental financial security measures.[16]

Age-appropriate services

Having age-appropriate services is a concern for most spouses, who think that day programs and nursing homes do not meet the needs of their physically strong and active spouses. This area is complex to address, because it is difficult to provide age-appropriate care for a small number of people who are usually not geographically concentrated. However, there are ways to integrate younger people into existing day programs and nursing homes. For example, the Samuel Lunenfeld adult day program at Baycrest Health Sciences in Toronto, Ontario, provides extra staffing and collaborates with the Sam and Ida Ross Memory Clinic to offer tailored day programming for younger people with frontotemporal dementia (FTD).[25] Clients participate in daily activities focused on behavior management, safety, hygiene, nutrition, mental health, creative expression, social and cognitive stimulation, and physical activity. This integrated, interdisciplinary approach ensures that the various health professionals treating a client with FTD share observations and expertise effectively and adjust care based on the combined knowledge and recommendations of neurologists, social workers, and nurses. The model alleviates the additional burden on caregivers to relay information from professional to professional.

For residential care, a similar model could be applied, in which a few facilities within each catchment area could have smaller units for people with YOD and in which specially trained staff can be provided to care for the younger, more mobile patients.

In-home supports

Respite and care in the home, with someone trained to deal with the behavioral and management issues of YOD, is needed to provide spouses with support and relief. In Ontario, in-home support is provided, free of charge, by a provincial government agency whose mandate is to provide care in the home. Their present criteria for offering in-home help are based on functional ability and memory (eg, need assistance with bathing, dressing, banking, housekeeping), which are areas that may not be impaired in some patients with YOD, but their judgment and lack of insight puts them at risk. Agencies that offer home-based supports should accommodate people who may not require assistance with activities of daily living but require staff to keep them engaged and safe while providing meaningful activities (eg, going for walks).

Health care system

A major obstacle in the health care system is the lack of information about YOD among health care professionals at all levels of practice.[1,4,22,23] Education is crucial and this is particularly important for acute care hospitals, in which spouses disproportionately (compared with their LOD counterparts) encounter vexing errors of provider judgment (eg, not realizing that the patient has a dementia and leaving them unattended, or assuming that the patients are competent to make their own health care decisions).[16] In Ontario, some hospitals have geriatric teams designed to intervene in the emergency department to advocate and educate staff around the needs of older adults and patients with dementia. However, because patients with YOD are less than 65 years of age, they cannot access these specialized services. A simple solution would be to accept younger patients with dementia to these specialized teams.

Another area of improvement would be to treat the patient-caregiver dyad as 1 unit of assessment and treatment, rather than just assessing the patient. When a patient with YOD comes for the first time to a specialized memory clinic the families should also be assessed to determine whether there is need for intervention. In this manner, caregivers could be proactively screened for depression and caregiver stress. Other areas that need to be addressed at this initial meeting include financial and legal planning issues, and assistance related to parenting children, who now will have to adapt to having a parent affected by YOD. In addition, patients and their spouses may need help in dealing with their own parents who are aging and may increasingly need support. Caregivers who are having difficulties should be offered interventions from the beginning to mitigate further problems.

Government/insurance programs

Young families who are affected by YOD are at a financial disadvantage, especially persons with YOD who do not have long-term disability or who are fired from their jobs (which excludes them from unemployment benefits). In addition, some well spouses may be forced to reduce or stop work in order to provide care.[15,16]

To address these issues, suggestions for financial aid include providing more hours of home help for those spouses who need to work outside the home, and eliminating or subsidizing the cost for day programs and respite services. In Ontario, those less than 65 years of age with acquired brain injuries or psychiatric conditions and individuals with developmental delays may qualify for free day programs and respite services, whereas there are no comparable programs for neurodegenerative diseases. More funds should be allocated to the underserved YOD population so that they can also have access to comparable services.

Another point to consider is that many countries in Europe already have in place a salary for caregivers as remuneration for their work.[26,27] This system has the benefit of allowing patients to be cared for at home for longer, while ensuring a modicum of financial support for families (because there is an increased risk of poverty for carers).[27]

Advocacy through education In order to advocate clinicians must first educate both professionals and the public about YOD.

The first step is to develop knowledge transfer strategies. It is necessary to create educational interventions at all levels, including health care, social service agencies, and government, which includes curricula development both at the postsecondary level and training of professionals at places of employment. In addition, university affiliates and organizations whose purpose is to translate research into practice could be enlisted to disseminate information. In addition, knowledge transfer needs to occur at the public level, which could be organized through organizations such as the Alzheimer societies (The Association for Frontotemporal Degeneration, CurePSP, the Creutzfeldt-Jakob Disease Foundation, and others), whose missions are to increase awareness and advocate for illnesses that cause YOD.

Micro Level of Intervention: Clinical/Community Engagement

Systemic and structural changes occur slowly; in contrast, clinical interventions can be more rapidly implemented by the clinicians and community agencies serving this population.

There is some evidence that psychotherapeutic and case management interventions are effective in reducing caregiver symptoms in spouses of individuals with LOD[12]; however, there is less evidence with regard to effective YOD caregiver interventions. The few YOD interventional studies focus on psychoeducational support groups[28–31] and respite care in combination with caregiver education and support.[32,33] These studies have shown reduction in caregiver burden and improved quality of life.

Interventions are needed that help spouses with their sense of isolation, depression, feelings of being misunderstood, and feelings of not being in control. The literature identifies group-based interventions to be effective.[16,30] One particular study, in which spouses of patients with YOD participated in a weekly online group,[30] found the online venue to be invaluable because it was easily accessible, it built community, and it was educational and supportive. This medium is a cost-effective way to provide psycho-therapeutic support, it is efficacious, and it can meet spouses' needs.[16,30]

PROPOSED INTERVENTIONAL STRATEGIES AT THE CLINICAL AND COMMUNITY LEVELS

Suggested forms of interventions discussed here are based on the dementia care-giving literature and my clinical and research experience.

Leisure Activities Groups

There is evidence in the LOD literature pointing to the effectiveness of leisure-based groups for caregivers that provide recreational and social opportunities.[34–36] Because spouses of patients with YOD have few opportunities for pleasurable activities, this could be a helpful intervention. Enjoyable activity-based groups could include walking clubs, bowling leagues, going to movies, and doing recreational and interactive pas-times that are normal for this group of people.

Telephone Support

Telephone support is another form of intervention, and has the advantage of not requiring scheduled visits to an office or center. There is a growing body of literature about the effectiveness of telephone-based psychotherapy.[37] Treatment barriers caused by the lack of time common to YOD caregivers suggest that telephone inter-ventions may be an efficient and effective mental health resource for this population. In addition to being a viable method to overcome caregivers' barriers to intervention, psychotherapy by telephone can be a valuable vehicle to help caregivers achieve a sense of control and mastery and, as Mozer and colleagues[37] put it, "facilitate resolu-tion or remission of psychiatric disorders, prevent symptom relapse, and supplement medical care in general." There is also evidence that a telephone-based intervention model that helps caregivers by providing information about available resources and emotional support is effective in reducing caregiver strain and increasing satisfaction with health care services and decreased hospital and emergency department use.[38] It is also my clinical experience that spouses find telephone interventions to be benefi-cial in decreasing anxiety by having someone to call for advice/support at the time that is needed, rather than waiting until a scheduled appointment, by which time the issue may no longer be relevant. Although providing psychosocial support via the telephone has limitations[39] (eg, professional liability for a client's safety, provision of psychother-apy to someone residing in a state other than that in which the therapist is licensed, and confidentiality), for this population it may be a viable approach given the dearth of resources. Spouses find that having a contact person to call with questions is help-ful and reassuring.

Capacity Building

First, given that spouses are isolated and need a supportive network and a sense of community, teaching people how to develop these networks is important. Drentea and colleagues[40] (2006) developed an effective intervention model that helped Alzheimer spousal caregivers mobilize their social support networks. Although the demonstration that this intervention model was effective focused on LOD spouses, it may have similar results with younger spouses. Furthermore, involving the family of origin at the point of diagnosis would be beneficial, because the loss of family support at this crucial time seems to be pervasive.[16] If families are included from the beginning and they have an opportunity to learn about the dementia and its effect on them, they may be more likely to be involved from the earlier stages. The same applies to family friends, who could join family meetings and could participate in the network of support.

A second area of capacity building is through social workers counseling spouses of patients with YOD on the importance of financial planning, powers of attorney, and where to obtain information and support related to financial and legal concerns.

Third, spouses report that health care providers tell them to take care of themselves, but they provide no guidelines on how to do this. As a way of intervention, professionals could help spouses compile a list of meaningful activities that bring them pleasure and remind them of the importance of self-care, which would help people expand their self-care repertoires. **Box 1** lists various self-care activities that were helpful to YOD spousal caregivers in my study (Shnall,[16] 2015).

Fourth, spouses want to preserve a sense of couplehood through the disease progression. One way to assist couples with this is by helping them create a repertoire of activities to be performed together, much like the list of self-care activities. Because there is evidence of the benefit of physical activity (improvement of overall physical health and mental, emotional, and social well-being)[41] for both partners, I have recommended to couples joint activities, which include physical exercise (**Box 2**). For

---

Box 1
Self-care activities for YOD spousal caregivers

- Sleep when tired and take advantage of times when partner is not home or is sleeping
- Make exercise part of a daily routine
- Eat healthy meals and snacks
- Build in personal time by getting up an hour earlier than spouse
- Schedule time with family and friends to talk and visit
- Laugh and see the humor in things
- Listen to sounds that bring pleasure (birds, music)
- Stretch
- Eat a favorite snack
- Hold hands or anything that brings basic human contact
- Read a quick magazine or something of interest
- Walk, enjoy the outdoors
- Journal
- Walk the dog
- Take pictures
- Cook a favorite meal
- Join a group (bowling, book club, cooking, running)
- Attend lectures, whether educational sessions at local Alzheimer societies or enjoyable lectures in the community
- Learn about something interesting
- Listen to podcasts
- Meditate and use mindfulness-based techniques regularly

Box 2
Tips on helping couples plan physical activities together

- Keep activities simple
- Physical activities should reflect what the person enjoys
- Provide positive reinforcement when the care recipient is performing an activity
- Some people may need assistance in choosing an activity or getting started
- Incorporate physical activities that both partners enjoy and try to do them regularly at the same time of day
- Individualized activities should be tailored to both partners' abilities
- Spend time outside doing these activities if possible
- There is an association between greater involvement of caregivers and greater care recipient participation in exercise

---

example, one couple enjoyed walking in the woods together and they had traveled the world hiking. When we met for the first time, it was evident that the caregiving spouse was missing this. Because the wife was now worried about her husband getting lost or losing interest in hiking for long periods of time, I suggested they resume hiking, but keep it shorter and closer to home, and that the client supervise her husband closely. As an added safety measure, her husband carries his cell phone, which has a GPS (global positioning system) application. With another couple I recommended doing stationary cycling at the local gym, because this form of exercise is safe (ie, people cannot get lost or lose their balance and fall off the bike), does not require much skill, and can be a fun group activity.

EFFECTIVE POINTS OF INTERVENTION: WHEN TO INTERVENE

The stage of the disease trajectory has consequences for the caregiving career.[16,42] In the early phases, when people are not ready to hear that their partner has a dementia, certain interventions are unlikely to be effective. For example, it would be difficult to offer day programs and counseling to spouses who do not believe that their partners have a dementia. What would be helpful at this point is to meet for a baseline assessment and to establish rapport, so that, when a crisis occurs, the spouse knows who to call. It would also be appropriate to offer one-on-one supportive counseling at this stage if the spouse feels ready. For those spouses who have suspected problems for a long time and are relieved to find out the cause, this would also be a good time to provide counseling.

Other transitions points that are important times for intervention are the loss of a job, loss of driving privileges, or Child Protective Services involvement, which are common problems for those affected by YOD.[18,43] Another transition point that necessitates intervention is the preadmission and admission process to residential care.[18] Spouses find this to be extremely difficult for several reasons. First, it is a separation of the couple as they know it and, although they may be ready for it, it is painful nonetheless. Second, spouses are usually in shock at the age of other residents and worry how their partners will fit in. Third, from a financial perspective, residential care is expensive and many families have to make painful financial sacrifices to pay for it. This transition point is an important time to discuss financial planning and budgeting priorities for these spouses, who will also have to secure their own financial futures. Fourth, spouses need to learn to trust the nursing staff and they need to find a balance between advocacy and forming alliances with these staff. Fifth, it is common for spouses to feel guilt and to believe that others will judge them harshly for placing their partners in residential care. In addition, because this is a time when spouses have more personal time after many years of caregiving, it is common for them to feel lost and to be unable to resume friendships or find new routines.

SUMMARY

There are 2 major proposed areas of intervention for those living with YOD. The first is at the macro level, dealing with the systemic barriers and gaps through education and advocacy, to avoid people failing to be helped by the social safety net. Not only should families affected by YOD have more access to services and resources but more comprehensive access to improved caregiver supports is a promising way to mitigate the growing economic burden of dementia. The second area of intervention is in the clinical and community areas of practice. At this level, knowing when it is an effective time to step in to help those living with YOD is as important as knowing how and what types of interventions are most effective. Supporting those living with YOD through public advocacy and community engagement leads to better psychosocial outcomes, thereby maintaining and improving their health and well-being.

REFERENCES

1. Bettie AM, Daker-White G, Gilliard J, et al. Younger people with dementia care: a review of service needs, service provision and models of good practice. Aging Ment Health 2002;6:205–12.
2. Shnall A, Agate A, Grinberg A, et al. Development of supportive services for frontotemporal dementias through community engagement. Int Rev Psychiatry 2013; 25:246–52.
3. Werner P, Stein-Shvachman I, Korczyn AD. Early-onset dementia: clinical and social aspects. Int Psychogeriatr 2009;2:631–6.
4. Van Vliet D, de Vugt M, Bakker C, et al. Impact of early-onset dementia on caregivers: a review. Int J Geriatr Psychiatry 2010;25:1091–100.
5. Svanberg E, Spector A, Stott J. The impact of young onset dementia on the family: a literature review. Int Psychogeriatr 2011;23:356–71.
6. Bakker C, de Vugt ME, van Vliet D, et al. The use of formal and informal care in early-onset dementia: results from the NeedYD study. Am J Geriatr Psychiatry 2013;21:37–45.
7. Shnall A. Supporting family caregivers of people with frontotemporal dementia. Can Rev Alzheimers Dis Dement 2009;12:14–6.
8. Arai A, Matsumoto T, Manabu I, et al. Do family caregivers perceive more difficulty when they look after patients with early-onset dementia compared to those with late-onset dementia? Int J Geriatr Psychiatry 2007;22:1255–61.
9. Harris PB. The perspective of younger people with dementia: still an overlooked population. Soc Work Ment Health 2004;2:17–36.
10. Zanetti O, Frisoni GB, Bianchetti A, et al. Depressive symptoms of Alzheimer caregivers are mainly due to personal rather than patient factors. Int J Geriatr Psychiatry 1998;13:358–67.
11. Freyne A, Kidd N, Coen R, et al. Burden in carers of dementia patients: higher levels in carers of younger sufferers. Int J Geriatr Psychiatry 1999;14:784–8.
12. Nunnemann S, Kurz A, Leucht S, et al. Caregivers of patients with frontotemporal lobar degeneration: a review of burden, problems, needs and interventions. Int Psychogeriatr 2012;24(9):1368–86.

13. Rosness TA, Mjorud M, Engedal K. Quality of life and depression in carers of patients with early-onset dementia. Aging Ment Health 2011;15:299–306.
14. Luscombe G, Brodaty H, Freeth S. Younger people with dementia: diagnostic issues, effects on carers and use of services. Int J Geriatr Psychiatry 1998;13: 323–30.
15. Hasse T. Early-onset dementia: the needs of younger people with dementia in Ireland. Dublin, Ireland: Alzheimer's Society of Ireland; 2005. Available at: http://www.alzheimer.ie/Alzheimer/media/SiteMedia/PDF's/Research/earlyOnsetDementia.PDF?ext=.pdf. Accessed November 25, 2014.
16. Shnall A. When least expected: stories of love, commitment, loss and survival – the experience and coping strategies of spouses of people with an early-onset dementia. Toronto (Canada): University of Toronto; 2015 [PhD thesis].
17. Van Vliet D, de Vugt M, Bakker C, et al. Time to diagnosis in young-onset dementia as compared with late-onset dementia. Psychol Med 2013;43:423–32.
18. Brodaty H, Donkin M. Family caregivers of people with dementia. Neuroscience 2009;11:217–28.
19. Cooper C, Katona C, Orrell M, et al. Coping strategies and anxiety in caregivers of people with Alzheimer's disease: the LASER-AD study. J Affect Disord 2006;90: 15–20.
20. Campbell P, Wright J, Oyebode J, et al. Determinants of burden in those who care for someone with dementia. Int J Geriatr Psychiatry 2008;23:1078–85.
21. Research. Rosalyn Carter Institute of Caregiving. Available at: http://www.rosalynncarter.org/evidence_based_resources/. Accessed November 22, 2014.
22. Roach P, Keady J, Bee P, et al. Subjective experiences of younger people with dementia and their families: implications for the UK research, policy and practice. Rev Clin Gerontol 2008;18:165–74.
23. Chemali Z, Schamber S, Tarbi EC, et al. Diagnosing early-onset dementia and then what? A frustrating system of aftercare resources. Int J Gen Med 2012; 5:81 6.
24. Raphael D. Tackling health inequalities: lessons from international experiences. Toronto (Canada): Canadian Scholars' Press; 2012.
25. Grinberg A, Phillips D. The impact of a community day program on the lives of patients with frontotemporal dementia and their caregivers. Can Rev Alzheimers Dis Dement 2009;12:17–22.
26. Social and welfare issues. Paris, France: Organization for Economic Cooperation and Development; 2014. Available at: http://www.oecd.org/social/. Accessed November 10, 2014.
27. Colombo F, Llena-Nozal A, Mercier J, et al. Help wanted? Providing for long-term care. Paris, France: Organization for Economic Cooperation and Development; 2011. Available at: http://www.oecd.org/els/health-systems/47884889.pdf. Accessed November 20, 2014.
28. Banks S, Rogalski E, Medina J, et al. Organizing a series of education and support conferences for caregivers of individuals with frontotemporal dementia and primary progressive aphasia. Alzheimers Care Q 2006;7:243–50.
29. Diehl J, Mayer T, Kurz A, et al. Features of frontotemporal dementia from the perspective of a special family support group. Nervenarzt 2003;74:445–9.
30. Marziali E, Climans R. New technology to connect frontotemporal dementia spousal caregivers online. Can Rev Alzheimers Dis Dement 2009;12(2):23–6.
31. Reah B, Julien C, Stopford C, et al. Developing a specialized support group for carers of people with frontotemporal dementia and semantic dementia. Dement Geriatr Cogn 2008;22:405–12.

32. Grinberg A, Lagunoff J, Phillips D, et al. Multidisciplinary design and implementation of a day program specialized for the frontotemporal dementias. Am J Alzheimers Dis Other Demen 2007;22:499–506.

33. Ikeda M, Imamura T, Ikejiri Y, et al. The efficacy of short-term hospitalizations in family care for patients with Pick's disease. Seishin Shinkeigaku Zasshi 1996; 98:822–9.

34. Bedini LA, Phoenix TL. Recreational programs for caregivers of older adults. In: Keller MJ, editor. Caregiving: leisure and aging. Binghamton (NY): The Hawthorne Press; 1999. p. 17–34.

35. Grosvenor BJ. Caregivers overlooked support: recreation therapy can help [Power Point Slides]. Available at: http://www.tbi-sci.org/conference/2012Presentations/Grosvenor-Caregivers_Recreation%20Therapy%20Feb%2024th.pdf. Accessed November 20, 2014.

36. Leitner M, Leitner S. Leisure in later life. 3rd edition. New York: Haworth Press; 2005.

37. Mozer E, Franklin B, Rose J. Psychotherapeutic intervention by phone. Clin Interv Aging 2008;3(2):391–6.

38. Bass DM. Care consultation telephone-based empowerment intervention. Americus, Georgia: Rosalyn Carter Institute of Caregiving; 2012. Available at: http://www.rosalynncarter.org/caregiver_intervention_database/. Accessed November 22, 2014.

39. Hass LJ, Benedict JG, Kobos JC. Psychotherapy by telephone: risks and benefits for psychologists and consumers. Prof Psychol Res Pr 1996;27:154–60.

40. Drentea P, Clay OJ, Roth DL, et al. Predictors of improvement in social support: five year effects of a structured intervention for caregivers of spouses with Alzheimer's disease. Soc Sci Med 2006;63:957–67.

41. Voss M, Nagmatsu L, Liu-Ambrose T, et al. Exercise, brain, and cognition across the life span. J Appl Physiol (1985) 2011;111(5):1505–13.

42. Nolan M, Lundh U, Grant G, et al, editors. Partnerships in family care: understanding the caregiving career. Maidenhead (United Kingdom): Open University Press; 2003.

43. Gibson MJ, Kelly KA, Kaplan AK. Family caregiving and transitional care: a critical review. San Francisco, California: Family caregiver alliance; 2012. Available at: https://caregiver.org/sites/caregiver.org/files/pdfs/FamCGing_TransCare_CritRvw_FINAL10.31.2012.pdf. Accessed November 15, 2014.

Index

Note: Page numbers of article titles are in **boldface** type.

Psychiatr Clin N Am 38 (2015) 363–371
http://dx.doi.org/10.1016/S0193-953X(15)00039-8
0193-953X/15/$ – see front matter © 2015 Elsevier Inc. All rights reserved.

psych.theclinics.com

Moving?

Make sure your subscription moves with you!

To notify us of your new address, find your **Clinics Account Number** (located on your mailing label above your name), and contact customer service at:

Email: journalscustomerservice-usa@elsevier.com

800-654-2452 (subscribers in the U.S. & Canada)
314-447-8871 (subscribers outside of the U.S. & Canada)

Fax number: 314-447-8029

Elsevier Health Sciences Division
Subscription Customer Service
3251 Riverport Lane
Maryland Heights, MO 63043

*To ensure uninterrupted delivery of your subscription, please notify us at least 4 weeks in advance of move.

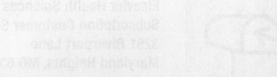

Printed and bound by CPI Group (UK) Ltd, Croydon, CR0 4YY

03/10/2024

01040494-0020